New Approaches to Disease, Disability, and Medicine in Medieval Europe

New Approaches to Disease, Disability, and Medicine in Medieval Europe

Edited by

Erin Connelly and Stefanie Künzel

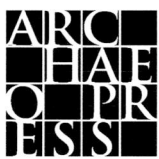

Archaeopress Publishing Ltd
Summertown Pavilion
18-24 Middle Way
Summertown
Oxford OX2 7LG

ISBN 978 1 78491883 5
ISBN 978 1 78491884 2 (e-Pdf)

© Authors and Archaeopress 2018

Cover illustration: St Roch, derived from Free Library of Philadelphia, MS Lewis E 175, fol. 116v

Digitized through Digitizing Hidden Special Collections and Archives, a Council on Library and Information Resources (CLIR) program generously supported by The Andrew W. Mellon Foundation

Project: Bibliotheca Philadelphiensis: Toward a Comprehensive Online Library of Medieval and Early Modern Manuscripts in PACSCL Libraries in Eastern Pennsylvania and Delaware

All rights reserved. No part of this book may be reproduced, or transmitted, in any form or by any means, electronic, mechanical, photocopying or otherwise, without the prior written permission of the copyright owners.

This book is available direct from Archaeopress or from our website www.archaeopress.com

Contents

Foreword 1
Christina Lee

Introduction 2
Erin Connelly and Stefanie Künzel

Þu miht wiþ þam laþan ðe geond lond færð: Conceptualisations
of Disease in Anglo-Saxon Charms 5
Stefanie Künzel

A Still Sound Mind: Personal Agency of Impaired People
in Anglo-Saxon Care and Cure Narratives 19
Marit Ronen

Mobility Limitations and Assistive Aids in the Merovingian
Burial Record 31
Cathrin Hähn

Tearing the Face in Grief and Rape: Cheek Rending
in Medieval Iberia, c. 1000–1300 43
Rachel Welsh

Clerical Leprosy and the Ecclesiastical Office:
Dis/Ability and Canon Law 62
Ninon Dubourg

Inside the *Leprosarium*: Illness in the Daily Life
of 14th Century Barcelona 78
Clara Jáuregui

Languages of Experience: Translating Medicine in MS Laud Misc 237 94
Lucy Barnhouse

Heillög Bein, Brotin Bein: Manifestations of Disease
in Medieval Iceland 109
Cecilia Collins

i

A Case Study of *Plantago* in the Treatment of Infected Wounds
in the Middle English Translation of Bernard of Gordon's
Lilium medicinae 126
Erin Connelly

Miserum spectaculum, horrendus fetor, aspectus horrendus: 'Syphilis' in
Strasbourg at the Turn of the 16th Century 141
Christoph Wieselhuber

Foreword

Christina Lee

Studies in Early Medicine is a peer-reviewed series designed to cover the growing discipline of the study of all aspects of disease, disability, health, medicine, and society in the ancient and early medieval world, from prehistory to the Middle Ages. Studies in Early Medicine is multidisciplinary as well as interdisciplinary and has welcomed papers from the fields of anthropology, archaeology, art, history, law, medicine and other studies related to medicine, health and society in the premodern past in diverse geographical areas.

Past volumes have arisen out of conferences and workshops devoted to specific themes. The present volume is devoted to the work of early career researchers and demonstrates how overarching themes of disability, disease, health, and medicine are relevant throughout premodern Europe from the Early Middle Ages up to the Renaissance.

Introduction

Erin Connelly and Stefanie Künzel

The majority of papers in this volume were originally presented at the eighth annual Disease, Disability, and Medicine in Medieval Europe conference (University of Nottingham, December 2014). The conference focused on infections, chronic illness, and the impact of infectious disease on medieval society, including infection as a disability in the case of visible conditions, such as infected wounds, leprosy, syphilis, and tuberculosis. Using an interdisciplinary approach, this conference emphasised the importance of collaborative projects, novel avenues of research for treating infectious disease, and the value of considering medieval questions from the perspective of multiple disciplines. Along those lines, colleagues from the field of microbiology presented papers on current work being done with quorum sensing, *Yersinia pestis*, climate and epidemics, and the efficacy of medieval medical recipes to treat modern infections. Essential to this discussion was a presentation of the results of a pilot study by Harrison *et al.* (mBio, 2015) on Bald's eyesalve (a 10th-century recipe contained in *Bald's Leechbook*, British Library Royal MS 12 D XVII). This work demonstrates the interdisciplinary applications of medieval medical questions and the great value of collaborative endeavours between the sciences and humanities.

The present volume aims to carry forward this interdisciplinary synergy by bringing together contributors from a variety of disciplines and from a diverse range of international institutions. Of note is the academic stage of the contributors in this volume. All of the contributors were PhD candidates at the time of the conference, and the majority have completed or are in the final stages of completing their programmes at the time of this publication. We hope the originality and calibre of research presented by these early career researchers demonstrates the promising future of the field, as well as the continued relevance of medieval studies for a wide range of disciplines and topics.

In addition to being diverse in discipline and location, the articles in this volume range from the beginning of the medieval period, with Anglo-Saxon and Merovingian topics, right up to the end of the 15th century. The articles are arranged chronologically.

The volume commences with 'Þu miht wiþ þam laþan ðe geond lond færð: Conceptualisations of Disease in Anglo-Saxon Charms', by Stefanie Künzel, which highlights how metaphoric thinking influenced the Anglo-Saxon expression of contagion in healing charms, particularly the 'Nine Herbs Charm'. Künzel reflects that former analyses of Anglo-Saxon medical texts often have been limited by modern assumptions about premodern medical competencies and, thus, significant information about perceptions of disease has been missed.

Along those lines, Marit Ronen presents a balanced consideration of the agency of impaired individuals in Anglo-Saxon society. In an examination of 119 cases from Anglo-Saxon narrative sources, 'A Still Sound Mind: Personal Agency of Impaired People in Anglo-Saxon Care and Cure Narratives', explores what can be learned about Anglo-Saxon societal expectations for an impaired person. Based on the case studies extant in the narratives, the chapter presents evidence to answer such significant questions as who was in charge of an impaired body and how much control did impaired persons have over their daily existence in Anglo-Saxon society.

Cathrin Hähn's chapter, 'Mobility Limitations and Assistive Aids in the Merovingian Burial Record', explores the significance of compensatory objects in Early Medieval burials in Germany and Switzerland. By comparing the numbers of relevant archaeological finds over the course of the medieval period as well as the materiality of the objects in question, Hähn comes to the conclusion that while objects such as prostheses and crutches are relatively rare in the burial record, the sophistication of their design suggests a development based on experience and usage.

In 'Tearing the Face in Grief and Rape: Cheek Rending in Medieval Iberia, c. 1000–1300', Rachel Welsh examines how the ritual of cheek rending used by women in medieval Iberia to mourn for the dead was also used as a legal requirement for proof of rape, according to the municipal lawcodes, *fueros*, of medieval Castile in the late 11th through the 13th centuries. In examining the practice of cheek rending as a bodily gesture with social, legal, and physical ramifications, this chapter analyses bodily mutilation as legal proof and considers the physical effects of cheek rending on the female body.

Using the *Decretals of Gregory IX*, canon laws, supplication letters, and papal dispensation letters, in 'Clerical Leprosy and the Ecclesiastical Office: Dis/Ability and Canon Law', Ninon Dubourg explores how the biblical label of 'unclean' was interpreted for 13th and 14th-century clerics who contracted leprosy. In light of this evidence, Dubourg considers the positive and negative social consequences for a medieval cleric diagnosed with leprosy.

Clara Jáuregui's 'Inside the *Leprosarium*: Illness in the Daily Life of 14th Century Barcelona' presents the first analysis of the account books (1379–1395) of the medieval leprosarium of Barcelona. Within the books is a wealth of information concerning the economic, religious, medical, and social circumstances of the leprosarium. This chapter brings attention and a new analysis to the operations and occupants of a hospital that has been largely forgotten in the historical record.

Lucy Barnhouse, in 'Languages of Experience: Translating Medicine in MS Laud Misc 237', explores a collection of eight medical texts which have not all been identified previously or examined as a group. Using clues found in the numerous marginal and interlinear notations, Barnhouse presents evidence to describe the 14th-century medical community that may have used these texts.

Cecilia Collins, in '*Heillög Bein, Brotin Bein*: Manifestations of Disease in Medieval Iceland', considers evidence of disease contained in textual sources in conjunction with the pathological samples of skeletal remains from church cemeteries and from the only known monastic hospital in Iceland (1493–1554), excavated at Skriðuklaustur (2002–2012). These records in both text sources and bone remains provide valuable insight into the prevalence of certain types of disease in medieval Icelandic society, as well as how care was provided in the community.

Erin Connelly, in 'A Case Study of *Plantago* in the Treatment of Infected Wounds in the Middle English Translation of Bernard of Gordon's *Lilium medicinae*', examines how medieval recipes used to treat infectious disease may inform modern antimicrobial research. Using medieval remedies from the 15th-century *Lylye of Medicynes*, Connelly explores the potential efficacy of *Plantago* spp. for wound healing and antimicrobial activity in light of present-day scientific studies.

To conclude the volume, Christoph Wieselhuber in '*Miserum spectaculum, horrendus fetor, aspectus horrendus*: "Syphilis" in Strasbourg at the Turn of the 16th Century', considers the social response to sexually-transmitted illnesses (referred to as *blattern, pocken,* or *syphilis*) through the lens of Johannes Geiler von Kaysersberg (1445–1510), an influential citizen of Strasbourg, who was 'the prince of the pulpit in the late 15th and early 16th centuries'.

The Institute for Medieval Research (University of Nottingham) and Universität Bremen were essential partners in the delivery of the Disease, Disability, and Medicine in Medieval Europe conference. A pre-conference postgraduate workshop was co-sponsored by the University of Nottingham and the Homo Debilis Creative Unit (Universität Bremen). The four sessions of the workshop led postgraduate students through the approaches (and problems) to researching medieval disease and disability from the perspectives of material culture, legal, historical, and literary positions. We would like to acknowledge Dr Christina Lee, University of Nottingham, who organised the conference and contributed the foreword as general editor. We extend special thanks to the University of Pennsylvania Libraries, Schoenberg Institute for Manuscript Studies for their support in the completion of this volume.

Þu miht wiþ þam laþan ðe geond lond færð: Conceptualisations of Disease in Anglo-Saxon Charms

Stefanie Künzel

The 'Nine Herbs Charm' is one of several metrical charms recorded in the *Lacnunga* ('remedies'), a collection of miscellaneous medical aids and prayers. It is transmitted in British Library Harley MS 585, fols. 130r–193r, an Anglo-Saxon compilation of medical texts dated to the late 10th or early 11th century. The current standard edition of the metrical charms was published in Elliott Van Kirk Dobbie's volume *The Anglo-Saxon Minor Poems*; another frequently quoted edition was produced by Grattan and Singer in 1952.

Given the context of the compilation in which the poem is transmitted, it has typically been recognised as a kind of healing charm. However, the details of the charm's linguistic design seem to position it closer to the genre of riddles than to that of medical recipes. As R. K. Gordon put it in his introductory statement to the Nine Herbs Charm, '[s]ome lines in this charm are now meaningless. It is clearly an old heathen thing which has been subjected to Christian censorship.'[1] While Gordon did not specify which lines he deems particularly alienating, he captures a common attitude towards Old English poetry, and the charms in particular, that has prevailed throughout most of 20th-century scholarship. He takes recourse to paganism—and the subsequent suppression of which—as an explanation for all things that do not make immediate sense within a modern framework of reference. I will argue that rather than being meaningless, the meaning of certain expressions is obscure to the modern interpreter but must have been meaningful within a contemporary model of thinking.

The aim of this essay is to investigate the meaning some of the words and expressions pertaining to the field of disease and healing might have had within their broader cultural context. The term *onflyge* ('on-flight' or, more commonly, 'on-flyers') and the phrase 'evil that travels across the land' (*laþan ðe geond lond færð*), both generally interpreted as referring to some sort of infectious disease, will be the focus of this investigation. It will be shown that such imagery is not merely a peculiar poetic device but reflects a common conceptualisation of disease in Anglo-Saxon times. On that basis, I suggest the 'Nine Herbs Charm' can be read

---

[1] Gordon (1954/1926: 92).

as an expression of deeply entrenched ways of thinking about disease, which shaped different methods of treatment in Anglo-Saxon England.

Already by the mid-19th century, the names of diseases had received attention within the broad discipline of Indo-European (or Indo-Germanic) studies. The mostly philological interest in the language of disease continued as one of the central lines of inquiry up until the 1940s.[2] From there onwards, disease came to be negotiated mainly in the form of histories of medicine as written by medics, not Anglo-Saxonists. The basic assumption underlying most of these publications is that medicine developed from archaic superstitious beliefs towards modern scientific insight.[3] Equipped with the latest knowledge about disease, scholars attempted to match medieval descriptions of disease with the nosological classifications of their own time. From that perspective, the medieval sources were characterised by omission of detail, confusion and distractions in the form of unscientific elaborations.[4] Coming from a background in social anthropology, Nigel Barley criticised earlier scholars for mistakenly overstressing historical origins of medical beliefs instead of looking at the synchronic system of approaching the issue of disease. This emphasis on historic views of disease and how they interact with methods of treatment marks a significant shift of focus.[5]

Another prevalent characteristic of the scholarship from the mid-20th century into the 1980s is a turn away from looking at disease in favour of analyses of medieval medical treatment of the latter. One of the paramount publications is Grattan and Singer's book *Anglo-Saxon Magic and Medicine: Illustrated specially from the Semi-Pagan Text 'Lacnunga'*. As a joint effort of a philologist and a historian of medicine with a background in science, it is an example of how knowledge of 20th-century medicine seems to have been viewed as a crucial prerequisite for anyone with the ambition of venturing into the diachronic study of disease and medicine. According to Charlotte Roberts, non–clinically trained researchers, especially anthropologists, were, in fact, actively discouraged from working in paleopathology.[6] In recent years, the study of medieval medicine has come to benefit from decidedly interdisciplinary efforts undertaken to prove that Anglo-Saxon medical recipes contain biomedically efficacious elements. One of the first researchers to give an optimistic appraisal of Anglo-Saxon medicinal treatments was Malcolm L. Cameron, who pointed out a number of ingredients, such as garlic and honey, that are still in use today and have been scientifically proven to be

---

[2] Cf. Geldner (1906); Lambert (1940); Pictet (1856).
[3] Cf. Bonser (1963). Winslow (1943).
[4] Brodman (1953: 267); MacArthur (1949, 1950, 1951); Shrewsbury (1949).
[5] Cf. Barley (1972: 68).
[6] Roberts (1998/2001: 1).

beneficial in cases of bacterial infection.⁷ Some doubt has since been cast upon Cameron's optimistic evaluation by a study claiming that some of the ingredients that individually have antibacterial properties are rendered useless when combined as prescribed.⁸ However, the latest results published by an interdisciplinary research group based at the University of Nottingham indicate the opposite of the earlier study's conclusions on the same recipe against eye infections transmitted in Bald's *Leechbook*.⁹

Nevertheless, in light of technological advances in genetics and microbiology that are starting to open up new directions of inquiry in the field of medieval studies, we are at danger of neglecting the value of textual sources. Under close examination, the linguistic evidence transmitted from the Anglo-Saxon period may offer a unique window revealing the different ways people might have thought about disease. Out of the entire corpus of Old English literature, only a small number of texts appear to be concerned with illness and healing to the same extent as the 'Nine Herbs Charm'. In that respect, it might prove particularly relevant in furthering our understanding of how conceptualisations of disease interrelate with methods of healing and illness prevention.

Cognitive approaches to literary interpretation of the texts produced in Anglo-Saxon England are just starting to be appreciated by researchers interested in gaining a better understanding of the mental processes at work behind medieval literature.¹⁰ Today, cognitive linguistics as well as cognitive poetics and cognitive cultural studies are cover terms for a variety of related approaches with more or less diverging orientations and interests. At the heart of these approaches lies a concern with language, the mind and culture.

Metaphors, accordingly, play a central role in the construction of reality. Yet, in some of the older studies on Anglo-Saxon disease and medicine, irrational language, such as expressions of metaphorical thought, was frequently lamented as a remainder of a pre-enlightened world of magic and paganism that distracts us from reality in the sense of absolute objective truth.¹¹ In considering metaphor not just as a stylistic device of poetic language, cognitive scientists distinguish between creative and conceptual metaphors. Creative metaphors are what most of us were trained to recognise as metaphors in English classes. Conceptual metaphors, on the other hand, are the very expressions of metaphoric thinking that pervade everyday language to such a degree that we all use them without even realising it

---

[7] Cameron (1982, 1983, 1993).
[8] Cf. Brennessel, Drout and Gravel (2005).
[9] Harrison *et al.* (2015).
[10] Gevaert (2005); Harbus (2012).
[11] Cf. Bonser (1963) and Winslow (1943), for example.

most of the time.[12] These conceptual metaphors have been holding a place at the core of cognitive linguistic research since the discipline was kick-started by the publication of George Lakoff's and Mark Johnson's *Metaphors We Live By* in 1980.

For the purpose of this essay, I would like to draw attention to one type of metaphor in particular—namely, what Lakoff and Johnson call ontological metaphors or entity metaphors.[13] Basically, they are ways of viewing events, activities, emotions, ideas, etc., as beings and substances. One example of viewing a nonphysical, abstract thing as an entity discussed by Lakoff and Johnson in *Metaphors We Live By* is INFLATION.[14] Conceptualising the experience of rising prices as an entity allows us to refer to it, quantify it, identify a particular aspect of it, see it as a causal agent and act with respect to it. One example, taken from the business section of the *New York Times*, would be the headline 'Asia tries to get a grip on inflation.'[15] Here, inflation is conceptualised as an object that can be physically held and potentially stopped. In another subcategory of ontological metaphors, the physical object is further specified as being an agent. Personification especially allows us to comprehend a wide variety of experiences with nonhuman entities in terms of human motivations, characteristics and activities.[16] This strategy can be illustrated with expressions like 'Inflation attacks the Dollar Menu'[17]—the headline of an article on how McDonalds cannot afford to offer burgers for the price of one dollar any longer. In this case, the metaphorical concept is not just INFLATION IS AN AGENT, but even more specifically INFLATION IS AN ADVERSARY.

In the following, I will show that some of the most basic yet pervasive metaphors pertaining to the concept of epidemic disease in the *Dictionary of Old English Corpus* are likewise entity metaphors/ontological metaphors; specifically, DISEASE IS AN ENTITY, DISEASE IS AN AGENT and DISEASE IS AN ADVERSARY.

The examples discussed below are the result of a digital search of the *Dictionary of Old English Corpus.*[18] The corpus has been searched for words meaning 'pestilence' or 'infection' according to the *Thesaurus of Old English* provided by the University of Glasgow.[19] The aim was to collect as many references to infectious or

---

[12] Lakoff and Johnson (1980: 3–6).
[13] Lakoff and Johnson (1980: 25–29).
[14] Capitalisation, in cognitive linguistic theory, is commonly used to denote the concepts and conceptual metaphors under discussion; I have adopted this practice.
[15] *New York Times*, 6 May 2008, viewed 30 August 2017 at <http://www.nytimes.com/2008/05/06/business/worldbusiness/06iht-rates.1.12605728.html>.
[16] Lakoff and Johnson (1980: 33–34).
[17] DailyReckoning.com, 29 October, viewed 30 August 2017 at < https://dailyreckoning.com/inflation-attacks-the-dollar-menu/>.
[18] Healey *et al.* (2000).
[19] University of Glasgow (n.d.).

even epidemic disease as possible in order to analyse the context of the individual occurrences for lexical, semantic or grammatical patterns. The collocation with verbs of motion as well as language pertaining to the semantic fields of battle and warfare turned out to be among the most salient features in the discourse of pestilence or, more neutrally speaking, infectious disease.

In Wulfstan's *Sunnudæges Spell*, *cwealm* is one of the punishments God is threatening to send over those who refuse to put down their work on Sunday: 'ic sende hæðen folc ofer eow, and þa eow benimað eowres eðles and eowres lifes; and ic sende on eowrum husum cwealm and hungor and untimnesse and fyr, þæt forbærnð ealle eowre welan'[20] ('I send heathens over you who shall take your possessions and your lives; and I send on your houses pestilence and hunger and misfortune and fire that shall burn all your riches'). *Cwealm* here is conceptualised as a thing or force under God's command that may be 'sent' to cause harm.

In other cases, pestilence is conceptualised as an agent of its own volition, as the following examples illustrate. In *De falsis diis*, one of Ælfric's homilies, 'com se cwealm sona and; mid færlicum deaðe þa philistheos acwealde'[21] ('soon came the pestilence and killed the Philistines with sudden death'). The same idea of the pestilence as an itinerant entity, physically moving around in space, is expressed in the poem 'Maxims I': 'Meotud ana wat hwær se cwealm cymeþ, þe heonan of cyþþe gewiteþ'[22] ('God alone knows where the pestilence goes that leaves here from our land'). In these examples, nouns denoting pestilence occur in close proximity with verbs signalling motion, *sendan* and *cuman*. In the former case, the disease is pictured as a passive entity controlled by another, specifically God, whereas the latter quotations point towards a conceptualisation of pestilence as an agent.

Other verb collocations include *forhergian* ('devastate') and *afligan* ('put to flight') which provide further evidence for disease being conceptualised as an enemy, specifically one encountered in the context of battle and warfare. We read of a 'cwylde, þe nu for þrym gærum þas ylcan burh forhergode mid swyþlicum wole 7 cwealme'[23] ('plague that for three years now has been devastating the same town with severe pestilence and death'). The verb *for-hergian* may be translated as 'to lay waste, destroy, ravage, devastate' or 'plunder'. It seems to be commonly used in contexts dealing with raiding armies as in 'Ceadwala eft forhergode Cent'[24] ('Ceadwalla again ravaged Kent') or 'her on þissum geare se cyning ferde

---

[20] HomU 35.1 (Nap 43), 67.
[21] ÆHom 22, 245.
[22] Max 1, 29.
[23] GDPref and 4 (C), 27.298.21.
[24] Chron A (Plummer), 687.1.

into Cumberlande and swiðe neah eall forhergode'[25] 'This year the king marched into Cumberland and destroyed [it] almost entirely'. In another example, a saint is asked that 'he his adl eallunge afligde'[26] ('put to flight his illness entirely'). This, once more, suggests the metaphor DISEASE IS AN ADVERSARY. Pestilence is characterised as an enemy that moves in space and may be 'put to flight' or 'driven away'. This last example especially conveys a sense of mobility of the intruding force that comes into a place from the outside with the intention to attack.

Notably, the 'Nine Herbs Charm' has not shown up in the results of my dictionary-based corpus-search. The words *cwealm* or *wol* are not used in the charm's description of the herbs' healing power. Nevertheless, some of the more obscure and seemingly rather poetic references to disease included in the charm can be understood as expressions of the same conceptual metaphors already encountered above: DISEASE IS A MOBILE ENTITY and DISEASE IS AN ADVERSARY.

The verse portion of the text appears much more elaborate in its composition than the brief lines of prose providing pointed instructions on how to prepare a medicine from the herbs listed. This formal separation has resulted in the text hardly ever being discussed as one coherent piece when it comes to its function and the rationale behind its composition.[27] In their prominent edition and translation, Grattan and Singer divide the charm into three parts and treat the prose recipe following the metrical section separately. In the translation, they title the first 29 lines 'Lay of the Nine Herbs', followed by the 'Lay of the Nine Twigs of Woden' (ll. 30–51) and the 'Lay of the Magic Blasts' (ll. 52– 63). For my analysis of expressions denoting disease, I am first going to focus on the beginning section of the charm, which below is reproduced in its entirety to give an impression of the general tone and structure of the piece. In the following, I will highlight rather smaller portions of text at the level of words and phrases which shall provide further evidence for the personification of disease throughout the 'Nine Herbs Charm'.[28]

      Gemyne ðu, mucgwyrt, hwæt þu ameldodest,
      hwæt þu renadest æt Regenmelde.
      Una þu hattest, yldost wyrta.
      ðu miht wið III and wið XXX,
5   þu miht wiþ attre and wið onflyge,

---

[25] ChronD (Classen-Harm), 1000.1.
[26] ÆCHom II, 10, 83.87.
[27] One recent exception may be found in Paz (2015), which investigates the integral role of poetry and language in medieval *scientia*.
[28] I have cited the Old English text after Dobbie's 1942 edition, which is also used in the *DOEC*; for comparison, see the translation by Grattan/Singer (1952).

þu miht wiþ þam laþan ðe geond lond færð.
　　　Ond þu, wegbrade, wyrta modor,
　　　eastan openo, innan mihtigu;
　　　ofer ðe crætu curran, ofer ðe cwene reodan,
10　　ofer ðe bryde bryodedon, ofer þe fearras fnærdon.
　　　Eallum þu þon wiðstode and wiðstunedest;
　　　swa ðu wiðstonde attre and onflyge
　　　and þæm laðan þe geond lond fereð.
　　　Stune hætte þeos wyrt, heo on stane geweox;
15　　stond heo wið attre, stunað heo wærce.
　　　Stiðe heo hatte, wiðstunað heo attre,
　　　wreceð heo wraðan, weorpeð ut attor.
　　　þis is seo wyrt seo wiþ wyrm gefeaht,
　　　þeos mæg wið attre, heo mæg wið onflyge,
20　　heo mæg wið ðam laþan ðe geond lond fereþ.
　　　Fleoh þu nu, attorlaðe, seo læsse ða maran,
　　　seo mare þa læssan, oððæt him beigra bot sy.
　　　Gemyne þu, mægðe, hwæt þu ameldodest,
　　　hwæt ðu geændadest æt Alorforda;
25　　næfre for gefloge feorh ne gesealde
　　　syþðan him mon mægðan to mete gegyrede.
　　　þis is seo wyrt ðe wergulu hatte;
　　　ðas onsænde seolh ofer sæs hrygc
　　　ondan attres oþres to bote.[29]

[29] [Have thou in mind, Mugwort, what thou didst reveal, / What thou didst establish at the mighty denunciation. / Una is thy name, oldest of herbs. / Thou art strong against three, and against thirty./5 Thou art strong against venom, and against the onflight / Thou art strong against that evil that fareth throughout the land. / And thou, Waybroad, mother of herbs ,/ From eastward open, mighty within. / Over thee have chariots rumbled, over thee have queens ridden, /10 Over thee have brides cried out, over thee have bulls snorted. / All didst thou then withstand and dost confound: / So do thou withstand venom and the onflight / And that evil thing that fareth throughout the land. / Stune is this herb named, on stone hath she grown. / 15 She standeth against venom, pain she assaulteth. / Stithe is her name, venom she confoundeth, / She driveth forth the evil things, casteth out venom. This is the herb which hath fought against snake. / This is strong against venom, she is strong against the onflight, / 20 She is strong against those evil things that fare throughout the land. / Rout thou now Attorlothe, the less rout the greater, / The greater the less, until to him be remedy from both. / Have thou in mind, Maythe, what thou didst reveal, / What thou didst bring to pass at Allerford, / 25 That never for flying ill did he yield up his life / Since for him Maythe was made ready for his eating. / This is the plant that Wergule is named, / This did the seal send forth over the high sea, / As cure for the wrath of

As pointed out above, questions of methods and instruments of curing, as well as of the curing agent, may shed some indirect light on the conceptualisation of disease. The 'Nine Herbs Charm' clearly merits some discussion of such questions. In the charm, several herbs are put forward for their usefulness against more or less specific afflictions. In that sense, one might interpret them as instruments of curing, as ingredients for remedies that need to be prepared and administered by someone—for example, a leech. Appropriate instructions on how to do that are provided in a prose section following the metrical section of the charm.

At the same time, the anonymous speaker's voice directly addresses some of the herbs by name and even explicitly reminds them of their function as contenders against disease. 'Gemyne ðu, mucgwyrt' (l. 1), 'Una þu hattest' (l.3), 'þu, wegbrade' (l. 7), 'attorlaðe' (l. 21), 'þu, mægðe' (l. 23). The herbs that are not addressed personally are 'stune' (l. 14), 'stiðe' (l. 16) and 'wergulu' (l. 27). What is interesting to note is how the line between the agent and the instrument working against a disease are blurred in case of the herbs which are listed as medical ingredients, while simultaneously being pitched as cognisant opponents to diseases.[30] The personification of plants by way of direct address may also be viewed as an indirect personification of the diseases they are supposed to cure.

With the actors of the charm identified, I will, once more, have a look at verbs. It will be shown that it is again the image of combat that best describes how herbs and disease are thought to interact, before analysing the specific characteristics of the afflictions targeted by the nine herbs. Two expressions in line 17, 'wreceð heo wraðan' ('she expels what is grievous/evil') and 'weorpeð ut attor' ('casts out poison'), could be seen as parallel constructions to 'he his adl eallunge afligde'. There is merely one instance of the word *gefeohtan*, meaning 'to fight', in line 18, while the phrase 'magan wið', 'to be strong, efficacious against', is employed several times (cf. ll. 4–6, 19–20). Just like the verb *wiðstandan* (ll. 11–12, 15–16), 'to stand against', it suggests resistance rather than action. The herbs in these cases would act more like a protective shield against attack as opposed to actively casting out invading forces that have already made it in. It appears that herbs work in different ways, perhaps depending on the kind of affliction they are meant to remedy.

I would now like to draw closer attention to the expressions 'onflyge' and 'laþan ðe geond lond fereþ', both of which have previously been understood as descriptions of infectious disease, although, it seems, rather intuitively.[31] In terms of conceptual metaphors, both fit the conceptualisation of DISEASE IS A MOBILE

---

another venom] (Grattan/Singer 1952).

[30] Cf. Paz (2015), section on the 'Nine Herbs Charm', especially p. 228.

[31] Cf. Barley (1972: 68).

ENTITY. The most obvious difference between the two would be the notion that one moves in the air while the other travels on land. Whereas *onflyge* may also express the idea of disease being an object that is in and transmitted via the air, another corresponding expression in the 'Nine Herbs Charm' is less ambiguous. A 'gefloge feorh', 'flying being or spirit' (l. 25), clearly indicates the conceptualisation of disease as an animated entity with the potential ability to move at will. The evil that wanders through the land, on the other hand, is characterised by the verb *faran,* which once again suggests purposeful movement. The underlying image might perhaps even be similar to those evoked by descriptions of human invaders as, for instance, 'se cyning ferde into Cumberlande and swiðe neah eall forhergode' discussed above.

Going back to the general distinction of flying and land-bound evils, another example, this time in prose form, shall serve to solidify the binary, but also, hopefully, illuminate their place within the broad category of afflictions a person might wish to protect oneself from. The following prose charm referred to as 'A Celestial Letter' is found in the 12th-century British Library MS Cotton Caligula A XV, fol. 140a.

> Se engel brohte þis gewrit of heofonum and lede hit on uppan Sanctus Petrus weofud on Rome.
>
> Se þe þis gebed singd on cyrcean, þonne forstend hit him sealtera sealma. And se þe hit singþ æt his endedæg, þonne forstent hit him huselgang.
>
> And hit mæg eac wið æghwilcum uncuþum yfele, ægðer ge fleogendes ge farendes.
>
> Gif hit innon bið, sing þis on wæter, syle hin drincan. Sona him bið sel. Gif hit þonne utan si, sing hit on fersce buteran and smere mid þæt lic. Sona him kymd bot.
>
> And sing þis ylce gebed on niht ær þu to þinum reste ga, þonne gescylt þe God wið unswefnum þe nihternessum on men becumað.[32]

---

[32] Cited after Storms (1948). [The angel brought this letter from heaven and laid it upon St. Peter's altar in Rome. He who sings this prayer in church will profit (as much) by it as by the psalms of the psalter. And to him who sings it on his death-bed it is equivalent to receiving the Eucharist. And it is also effective against every unknown evil either flying or traveling. If it is an inner (evil), sing this over water, give him to drink; soon he will be well. If it is an external (evil), sing it on fresh butter and smear his body with it; soon he will become healthy. And sing this same prayer at night before you go to your rest; then God will protect

The charm, sometimes called a prayer, is said to be effective against 'æghwilcum uncuþum yfele, ægðer ge fleogendes ge farendes'. The expression 'æghwilcum uncuþum' ('every/any unknown') suggests a degree of uncertainty about the exact nature of the evil in question. Even more striking is that the aspect that can be and is specified is the mode of movement. To take the description further, the evils are portrayed as affecting the body on the inside or the outside and therefore call for internal or external treatment. Again, disease is conceptualised as existing independent of a particular outbreak of illness in an individual; it can be in transit, so to speak. The apparent distinction between flying and wandering evils may be due to the perception of two separate diseases or disease-types that are conceptualised in partially similar ways (that is, mobile, but in different spheres of the environment) or may reflect two alternative conceptualisations of the same thing.

A very similar concept can be found in the so-called 'Journey Charm', another text typically included in the group of the metrical charms.

>   Ic me on þisse gyrde beluce and on godes helde bebeode
>   wið þane sara stice, wið þane sara slege,
>   wið þane grymma gryre,
>   wið ðane micela egsa þe bið eghwam lað,
> 5   and wið eal þæt lað þe in to land fare.
>   Sygegealdor ic begale, sigegyrd ic me wege,
>   wordsige and worcsige.³³

The expression 'eal þæt lað þe in to land fare' again implies an inside and an outside in relation to a certain physical space. The 'lað' is seen as coming into that area from some place not specified. The 'sore stitch' and the 'sore bite' could be the same thing or two variants of the same type of thing reminiscent of the *fær-stic* that gives the title to another charm in the *Lacnunga*.³⁴ The 'grymma gryre' and the 'micela egsa þe bið eghwam lað' might be paraphrases referencing the same concept. What that might be, however, remains unidentified. In terms of disease,

---

you from dreams and nightmares that come upon men.]

³³ Cited after Dobbie (1942). [I encircle myself with this twig and entrust myself to God's grace, against the sore stitch, against the sore bite, against the grim dread, against the great terror that is loathsome to everyone, and against all evil that travels into the land. A victory-charm I sing, a victory-twig I carry, word-victory and work-victory.]

³⁴ Heather Stuart also points out this parallel and suggests that 'færstice most probably refers to a form of elfshot which emerges physically as epidemic disease' (Stuart 1981: 266). However, she does not provide much of an explanation of how she gets to this particular conclusion.

the qualifier *micel* and the characterisation as potential harm to everyone ('bið eghwam lað') could be descriptive of an epidemic of some kind.

From the perspective of cognitive metaphor theory, the concept of epidemic disease would be grounded in experience. Such experiences might include the detection of symptoms in a considerable number of individuals up to virtually everyone. Coupled with the appearance of symptoms in different, perhaps geographically connected locations over an observable period of time, the characterisation as *micel* would be well motivated. The same observations could also be the motivation behind the conceptual metaphor DISEASE IS A MOBILE ADVERSARY of which I propose 'the evil that travels across the land' and 'the evil that comes into the land' to be expressions. Note that according to such a conceptualisation, disease is located not within the body itself but—while not symptomatic—in the outside world.

What has been detected is a binary conceptualisation of disease which prefigures a strategic combination of treatments. These entail, on the one hand, biomedically efficacious medicines against symptoms of illness manifest on the human body. They could, for instance, be administered in the form of salves and potions as evidenced in the Nine Herbs Charm's prose instructions for the preparation of an herbal remedy. Simultaneously, disease is imagined as existing apart from its concrete manifestations and symptoms, as a cognisant entity present in the environment. This entity is called out upon when singing a charm; it is urged to leave the patient or stay away in a prophylactic sense.

What this essay has been trying to highlight is the cognitive capacity of metaphoric thinking, common to all of humanity, which has informed how Anglo-Saxon people dealt with the realities of their environment, including disease. The different ways of thinking about and reacting to disease need not be regarded as a sign of confusion or be mutually exclusive but may effectively go hand in hand, as it has been exemplified in the 'Nine Herbs Charm'.

Bibliography

Banham, D. 2002. Investigating the Anglo-Saxon *Materia Medica*: Archeobotany, manuscript art, Latin and Old English, in R. Arnott (ed.), *The Archaeology of Medicine. Papers given at a session of the annual conference of the Theoretical Archaeology Group held at the University of Birmingham on 20 December 1998* (B.A.R. International Series 1046): 95–99. Oxford: Archeopress.

Banham, D. 2011. Dun, Oxa and Pliny the Great Physician: Attribution and authority in Old English medical texts. *Social History of Medicine* 24(1): 57–73.

Barley, N. 1972. Anglo-Saxon magico-medicine. *Journal of the Anthropological Society of Oxford* 3(2): 67–76.

Barney, S. A., Lewis, W. J. et al. 2006. *The Etymologies of Isidore of Seville.* Cambridge: Cambridge University Press.

Bonser, W. 1963. *The Medical Background of Anglo-Saxon England.* Oxford: Oxford University Press.

Bosworth, J. and Toller, T. N. 1898. *An Anglo-Saxon Dictionary.* Oxford: Clarendon Press.

Brennessel, B., Drout, M., and Gravel, R. 2005. A reassessment of the efficacy of Anglo-Saxon medicine. *Anglo-Saxon England* 34: 183–195.

Brodman, E. 1953. Medieval epidemics. *Bulletin of the Medical Library Association* 41(3): 265–272.

Cameron, M. L. 1982. The sources of medical knowledge in Anglo-Saxon England. *Anglo-Saxon England* 11: 135–155.

Cameron, M. L. 1983. Bald's Leechbook: Its sources and their use in its compilation. *Anglo-Saxon England* 12: 153–182.

Cameron, M. L. 1993. *Anglo-Saxon medicine.* Cambridge: Cambridge University Press.

Cockayne, O. 1865. *Leechdoms, wortcunning, and starcraft of early England.* London: Longman.

Crawford, S. and Randall, A. (2002). Archeology and documentary sources: Two Approaches to Anglo-Saxon medicine, in R. Arnott (ed.), *The archeology of medicine: Papers given at a session of the annual conference of the Theoretical Archeology Group held at the University of Brimingham on 20 December 1998* (B.A.R. International Series 1046): 101–104. Oxford: Archaeopress.

Crawford, S. and Lee, C. (eds) 2010. *Bodies of Knowledge: Cultural Interpretations of Illness and Medicine in Medieval Europe.* Oxford: Archaeopress.

Dobbie, E. V. K. (ed.) 1942. *The Anglo-Saxon minor poems.* New York: Routledge, Kegan Paul.

Geeraerts, D. and Grondelaers, S. 2009. Looking back at anger: Cultural traditions and metaphorical patterns, in D. Geeraerts (ed.), *Words and Other Wonders: Papers on Lexical and Semantic Topics:* 227–251. Berlin: Mouton de Gruyter. (Originally published in J. Taylor and R. E. MacLaury [eds], 1995. *Language and the Construal of the World:* 153–180. Berlin: Mouton de Gruyter.)

Geldner, J. 1906. *Untersuchung einiger altenglischer Krankheitsnamen.* Braunschweig: Westermann.

Gevaert, C. 2005. The anger is heat question: Detecting cultural influence on the conceptualisation of anger through diachronic corpus analysis, in N. Delbacque, J. Van der Auwera and D. Geeraerts (eds), *Perspectives on Variation: Sociolinguistic, Historical, Comparative:* 195–208. Berlin: de Gruyter.

Grattan, J. H. G. 1927. Three Anglo-Saxon charms from the 'Lacnunga'. *Modern Language Review* 22(1): 1–6.

Grattan, J. H. G. and Singer, C. 1952. *Anglo-Saxon magic and medicine: Illustrated specially from the semi-pagan text 'Lacnunga'*. London: Oxford University Press.

Harbus, A. 2012. *Cognitive Approaches to Old English Poetry*. Cambridge: D. S. Brewer.

Harrison, F., Roberts, A. E. L., Gabrilska, R., Rumbaugh, K. P., Lee, C., and Diggle, S. P. 2015. A 1000-year-old antimicrobial remedy with antistaphylococcal activity. *mBio* 6(4): e01129-15. doi:10.1128/mBio.01129-15.

Hays, J. 2007. Historians and epidemics: Simple questions, complex answers, in L. K. Little (ed.), *Plague and the End of Antiquity: The Pandemic of 541-750*: 33–58. Cambridge: Cambridge University Press.

Healey, A., Holland, J., McDougall, I., and Mielke, P. *The Dictionary of Old English Corpus in Electronic Form, TEI-P3 conformant version, 2000 Release* (CD-ROM). Toronto: DOE Project 2000.

Lakoff, G. and Johnson, M. 1980/2003. *Metaphors We Live By*. Chicago: University of Chicago Press.

Lambert, C. 1940. The Old English medical vocabulary. *Proceedings of the Royal Society of Medicine* 33: 137–145.

MacArthur, W. 1949. The identification of some pestilences recorded in the Irish annals. *Irish Historical Studies* 6: 169–188.

MacArthur, W. 1950. Comments on Shrewsbury's 'The Yellow Plague'. *Journal of the History of Medicine and Allied Sciences* 5(2): 214–215.

MacArthur, W. 1951. The pestilence called *scamach*. *Irish Historical Studies* 7: 199–200.

Meaney, A. L. 1992. The Anglo-Saxon view of the causes of illness, in S. Campbell, B. Hall and D. Klausner (eds), *Health, Disease and Healing in Medieval Culture*: 13–33. New York: St. Martin's.

Meaney, A. L. 2000. The practice of medicine in England about the year 1000. *Social History of Medicine* 13(2): 221–237.

Meaney, A. L. 2011. Extra-medical elements in Anglo-Saxon medicine, in *Social History of Medicine* 24(1): 41–56.

Paz, J. 2015. Magic that works: Performing *Scientia* in the Old English metrical charms and poetic dialogues of Solomon and Saturn. *Journal of Medieval and Early Modern Studies* 45(2): 219–243.

Pettit, E. 2001. *Anglo-Saxon Remedies, Charms, and Prayers from British Library MS Harley 585: The 'Lacnunga'*, 2 vols. Lewiston: Edwin Mellen Press.

Pictet, A. 1856. Die alten Krankheitsnamen bei den Indogermanen. *Zeitschrift für vergleichende Sprachforschung auf dem Gebiete des Deutschen, Griechischen und Lateinischen* 5(5): 321–354.

Roberts, C. 1998/2001. Paleopathology and archeology, in R. Arnott (ed.), *Archeology of Medicine. Papers given at a session of the annual conference of the Theoretical Archeology Group held at the University of Brimingham on 20 December 1998* (B.A.R. International Series 1046): 1–20. Oxford: Archaeopress.

Shrewsbury, J. F. D. 1949. The yellow plague. *Journal of the History of Medicine and Allied Sciences* 4(1): 5–47.

Storms, G. 1948. *Anglo-Saxon magic*. The Hague: Martinus Nijhoff.

Stuart, H. 1981. 'Ic me on þisse gyrde beluce': The structure and meaning of the Old English *journey charm*. *Medium Ævum* 50: 259–273.

Talbot, C. H. 1967. Some notes on Anglo-Saxon medicine. *Medical History* 9: 156–169.

Roberts, J. and Kay, C. with Grundy, L. n.d. *A Thesaurus of Old English,* University of Glasgow, viewed 30 August 2017 at <http://oldenglishthesaurus.arts.gla.ac.uk/>.

Van Arsdall, A. 2005. Reading medieval medical texts with an open mind, in E. Lane Furdell (ed.) *Textual Healing: Essays on Medieval and Early Modern Medicine*: 9–29. Leiden: Brill.

Winslow, C. E. A. 1943. *The Conquest of Epidemic Disease: A Chapter in the History of Ideas.* Princeton (NJ): Princeton University Press.

A Still Sound Mind: Personal Agency of Impaired People in Anglo-Saxon Care and Cure Narratives

Marit Ronen

The question of agency of impaired people is an important and often opaque one in Medieval Disability Studies, yet it is a foundational issue. External control over the bodies of impaired people (expressed most directly through care and cure processes) is fundamentally othering, as well as contributing to the constructions of weakness, dependence, and disability. A feeling of powerlessness, especially over one's own body, is a central aspect of oppression.[1] The physical realities of Anglo-Saxon England made the need for physical help and care a pivotal part of the lives of impaired people, and their representation in narrative sources.[2] Yet the equation of physical help with dependency, and of dependency with a lack of agency, was not as central in Anglo-Saxon perceptions of impairment and disability, as it is today.

    Anglo-Saxon sources show a spectrum of agency in narratives of the lives, care, and cure of impaired people. Like many other medieval societies, Anglo-Saxon England did not produce many sources from the point of view of impaired people and rarely made an effort to represent their experiences (some texts were written by impaired individuals, but do not contain information on their lived experiences), and in most narrative sources impaired people were objects upon which outside forces acted. This can give the impression of passivity and lack of agency, but closer examination of the roles filled by impaired people in the sources reveals complex cultural attitudes which often accepted, and even expected, the agency of impaired people. While political and economic agency is evident in many of those, at the basis of questions of agency is control of one's own body. I will attempt to shed some light on this essential issue through an examination of a specific kind of agency in Anglo-Saxon sources. Specifically, I will discuss perceptions regarding the ability of impaired people to direct their own care (or that of others) and to make decisions regarding their conditions and fate. This can be expressed both through physical actions and, importantly, through constructions of authority. The level of involvement in, and control of, the care and cure of impaired people

---

[1] Wilkerson 2002, 41-42.
[2] Lee 2012, 27-29.

is not always easily detected. It requires reading between the lines and reliance on incidental information. Most sources presented impaired people with agency: of the 119 cases in the narrative sources which contain some information regarding the level of agency, 83 contain evidence of agency in care and cure, and 36 contain evidence of a lack of agency (out of which 17 are of impaired children).

Agency in care and cure narratives

There was a certain youth, a paralytic, who was brought in a wagon from another monastery to the skilled physicians of our monastery [Lindisfarne]. They began to try every cure on him as he lay with almost all his limbs mortified and powerless. After toiling long, they had no success and gave him up altogether, despairing of curing him. When the boy saw himself deserted by human doctors, he said to his servant with lamentations and tears: 'This powerlessness and mortification first began from my feet and so spread through all my members. So I ask the abbot for the shoes which were on the feet of the holy and incorruptible martyr of God [Cuthbert].' According to his counsel, the servant brought the shoes and he put them on his feet that night and rested.

> Fuit namque quidam adolescens paraliticus de alio monasterio in plaustro deductus ad medicos edoctos cenobii nostri. Illi enim onmi cura eum qui pene cunctis membris mortifactis dissolutus iacebat, medere ceperunt, nihilque proficientes, post longum laborem omnino deseruerunt, disperantes curare eum. Puer itaque desertum se a medicis carnalibus ut uidit, plorans et lacrimans ministro suo dixit, Primum utique mihi hoc malum desolutionis et mortificationis inchoans a pedibus per omnia membra deseminauit. Ideo namque deposco ab abbate calciamenta quo circumdederunt pedes sancti martyris Dei incorruptibilis, et secundum consilium eius ficones detulit, pedibus suis nocte illa circumdedit, et requieuit.[3]

This youth was able to choose a correct course of action (while experts failed to do so), commanded others to assist him, and explained the logic beyond his actions (he requested Cuthbert's shoes because his impairment originated in his feet). By doing that, the youth displayed a high level of personal agency and control of his situation in life, despite the many social factors that could have prevented it – his subordination to a monastic hierarchy, his age, and his physical condition. In the end, his personal agency, his control of himself, won out.

---

[3] Anonymous Monk of Lindisfarne 1969, 136-139.

Often agency of impaired people was illustrated by their ability to plan a course of action, to act to elevate their condition, and to direct others in assisting them. Christina Lee has already pointed out that by seeking the help of others, impaired people were agents in their own cure narratives.[4] In these narratives, the authors both acknowledge the reality of physical dependence (common to many Medieval impaired people) and detached from the body the question of agency over the body. While the agency of impaired people has often been viewed in terms of physical dependence or independence, Disability Studies have rather emphasised decision-making as a crucial element. Additionally, within cultural understandings of people as vulnerable and interdependent, the notion of physical reliance on others need not necessarily translate to diminished agency.[5] In the following discussion, the idea of physical dependency as unconnected with, or as not damaging of, personal agency will come to the fore.

Three versions of the *Life of Swithun* tell of a paralysed, bed-ridden man, who heard of the miracles performed by Swithun. Lantfred wrote how he 'began to consider in his still sound mind' [*coepit sagaci mente praemeditari*] that he should visit the saint's tomb, and so 'urged' [*precepit*] his kin to take him there.[6] Wulfstan of Winchester emphasised the man's physical weakness and need of assistance, but still had him summon his kin and direct their actions.[7] Even the Miracula S. Swithuni, which had the man 'humbly ask[ing]' [*humiliter rogat*] for his kin's help, portrays him as directing their actions.[8] The relationship between physical dependency and mental agency is here highlighted. While the man is clearly (and increasingly) presented as physically dependent on the help of his kin, he always remains in control of the situation, able to make decisions and direct others. In the three versions, even when the man's physical limitations were emphasised, the initiative and the final decision regarding his care were his.

A similar reliance on physical help while maintaining agency can be found in a second episode from Lantfred. An impaired man's friends and family could not find a cure for him, or a doctor to treat him, and in their desperation, they suggested a pilgrimage to Saint Iudoc's tomb. The man agreed and arranged for the trip, but in the night, he had a vision directing him to go to Saint Swithun's tomb instead. When his friends returned, he informed them of his change of plans, and was led by them to Saint Swithun's tomb, where they waited outside while he

---

[4] Lee 2012, 27-29.
[5] Reindal 1999, 353, 364.
[6] Lantfred of Winchester 2003, 291.
[7] Wulfstan of Winchester 2003, 469-471.
[8] 'Miracula S. Swithuni' 2003, 655.

held a vigil throughout the night.⁹ While this man relied on his friends and family to seek medical care for him, and then to assist him in his pilgrimage, he was clearly in control of the situation: his approval was needed in order to abandoned medical solutions and turn to religious ones, and it was his decision when to go on pilgrimage and to where – much like Cuthbert's paralytic youth, he was able to choose a correct course of action, while others stirred him wrong. His hale peers were not able to direct his care as well as he was.

The various versions of the *Life of Swithun* contain several more cases of rivalry between shrines and competition for pilgrims. They include impaired people deciding where to go (be it a correct or incorrect decision) without the counsel or direction of other people, expected to be in control of their care and cure, even when the wrong course of action was decided upon, without any doubt cast by the authors on their ability to make decisions or to exercise agency.¹⁰

A further example from the *Life of Swithun* will illustrate this point more clearly. A *materfamilias* suffered from an unidentified illness and vowed to give gifts to Saint Swithun's shrine if she was healed. However, after being healed 'she apparently lost her mental faculties since [...] she did not fulfill the promises to which she had committed herself'. [*amisit uigorem mentis, quoniam [...] promissiones quibus sese obligauerat non obseruauit et gratias Deo debitas (sicut condignum erat) non rependit.*] She relapsed, recognised her mistake, repented and was again healed.¹¹ While ill, the woman was capable of making a vow, demonstrating her mental faculties on which doubt was cast only when, in health, she failed to fulfill her promise. As mental ability was so central to constructions of impaired people's agency, this is a fascinating description - highlighting not only the woman's abilities while ill, but also positioning them as greater than when healthy. The impression created is of better decision-making skills accompanying illness.

Additionally, the woman's husband was mentioned only off-handedly in both versions of the story, and all actions in the story, for better or worse, were performed by the woman, which demonstrates how agency in care and cure was not reserved only for men. While I will shortly show how subordinate social positions could impact impaired people's agency, it is interesting that, as shown here, gender was not always one such factor.

---

⁹ Lantfred of Winchester 2003, 279-281; Ælfric 1966, 66.
¹⁰ For example, see Wulfstan of Winchester 2003, 547; Lantfred of Winchester 2003, 297 (repeated in Wulfstan of Winchester 2003, 481-483; 'Miracula S. Swithuni' 2003, 659), and Lantfred of Winchester 2003, 299 (repeated in Wulfstan of Winchester 2003, 485-487; 'Miracula S. Swithuni' 2003, 659-661).
¹¹ Lantfred of Winchester 2003, 291-293, repeated in Wulfstan of Winchester 2003, 471-475.

Some examples deal with impaired individuals who were helped by clearly subordinate people. The paralysed boy, mentioned at the opening of this section, is one such example, commending as he did a servant to fetch him Cuthbert's shoes. Also in the *Life of Saint Cuthbert*, a priest from Willibrord's monastery came to Lindisfarne, and there fell mortally ill. '[T]hinking of a profitable plan' [*inuento salubri consilio*],[12] he instructed his servant to lead him to the church where Cuthbert was buried and was there healed. Similarly, in *De Abbatibus*, a severely ill monk who could not move, only speak, commanded a servant to bring him a holy relic, and was cured.[13] This monk, presented as completely physically disabled (apart from speech), was nonetheless able to direct his care and command others. The theme of dependence versus authority which emerges is, I posit, the very root of impaired people's agency in these narratives.

Cuthbert himself, while dying of an illness, chose an old monk who suffered from chronic dysentery to remain with him and care for him (a great honour).[14] Here are demonstrated both Cuthbert's agency in arranging his care, and the agency of the old monk, Walhstod, who was perceived as able to care for the dying saint – and thus, presumably, for himself as well. *The Life of St. Cuthbert* by Bede does not mention Cuthbert's selection, but does include Walhstod and his old age and illness.[15] Although Walhstod did not choose his own course of action, underlain here is the assumption that he was able to arrange and provide care.

A special category of agency in care and cure narratives is that of visions, which can both contribute to the agency of impaired individuals, and to their alienation: on the one hand, they are an expression of a close connection with the divine and give a special authority to the people having them, but, on the other hand, such connections between impairment and divinity are often interpreted, with merit, as instances of the 'super-crip' topos, and as contributing to the othering and alienation of impaired people.[16]

For the purpose of this article, it is the authority derived from visions which will be of interest. Whether or not they could cause or enhance social isolation, they consistently imbued vision recipients with power over themselves and others. A good example is found in the *Life of Edward Martyr*: a matron with severely crushed feet had a vision in which the martyred King Edward instructed her to go to his tomb. However, when in the morning she shared her vision with her neighbours, she was convinced by them that it was not real and did nothing.

---

[12] Bede 1969b, 297.
[13] Æthelwulf 1967, 20.
[14] Anonymous Monk of Lindisfarne 1969, 129.
[15] Bede 1969b, 271.
[16] Bragg 1997, 165-166, 170.

She then had a second vision, in which Edward chastised her because she did not follow his instructions and again told her to visit his tomb. This time the woman obeyed, went to Edward's tomb, and was healed.[17] The play of agency and authority is clear – the neighbours, speaking against the vision and against the matron's authority regarding her own condition, were mistaken, and the matron's agency was validated.

The insistence on the authority of the vision recipient, even if impaired, is articulated in the *Life of Edward the Confessor*: as the king lay dying, he had a vision of the conquest of England by the Normans. But hearing it, Archbishop Stigand rejected it, saying Edward was 'broken with age and disease and knew not what he said.' [*senio confectum et morbo, quid diceret nescire*]. His denial of the king's vision was proven to be a mistake, and the king's authority (and that of his vision) upheld, regardless of his illness.[18]

Visions crossed gender and status boundaries. A young woman with an infection in her throat, as well as three blind men, all had visions instructing them to go to King Edward the Confessor.[19] The various lives of Saint Swithun include a smith, the man whose friends suggested a pilgrimage to Saint Iudoc, as well as of a paralysed man who had an elaborate vision of Saint Swithun, and was healed after visiting his tomb.[20] A blind man,[21] a woman with a heart condition,[22] and the paralysed Abbess Aelfflaed[23] further demonstrate how impaired people of all genders and walks of life were portrayed as able to receive visions regarding their situations, and to exercise their agency.

Through all these examples of representations of the agency of impaired people, their mental abilities, as existing regardless, and detached from, physical dependency, were emphasised. However, the common reliance on physical assistance in the sources also often created an impression of a lack of agency – certainly in the minds of modern readers.

Lack of agency in care and cure narratives

Examples of a lack of agency can be largely divided into three groups: of 37 examples, 22 were based on ambivalent lexical evidence (some of which were also

---

[17] Edward King and Martyr 1971, 11.
[18] The Life King Edward Who Rests at Westminster 1992, 118/119.
[19] Ibid, 93, 95, 97.
[20] Wulfstan of Winchester 2003, 539-545, repeated in 'Miracula S. Swithuni' 2003, 673-675.
[21] Wulfstan of Winchester 1991, 65.
[22] Aldhelm 2009, 121.
[23] Bede 1969b, 233.

of children), 17 were of children (lacking agency based on that fact alone), and five were of people in subordinate positions, yielding to authority.

The nature of the sources dictated a passive role for impaired people, as objects upon whom saints acted. Passive language was also commonly used and contributed to this impression: relatives took and led [*deducunt and adducunt*] a woman to Saint Swithun,[24] and a sick man's friends wanted to carry him [*ferian*] to Winchester.[25] Verbs such as *perductum*,[26] *deducitur*,[27] *ducitur*,[28] *deducta*,[29] *fertur*,[30] *defertur*,[31] *positus*[32] and *geboren*[33] are just a few examples. This use of passive language to describe the impaired person's involvement in the care and cure process can be taken to reflect wider attitudes regarding lack of agency. At the same time, they could be generic choices which obscured a more active involvement by impaired people.

The dangers of assuming passivity are made clear by several examples in the sources. A paralysed man heard of the miracles performed by Saint Swithun and decided to hold a vigil at his tomb, and depended on his kin and neighbours for help in getting to Winchester;[34] a very sick man asked his friends to take him to Winchester;[35] a blind man went to Winchester, 'follow[ing] the advice of his friend and his own inclination' [*suo et amicorum consilio*];[36] a paralysed man 'was taken – in accordance with his wishes – by his kinsmen to Winchester' [*ab agnatis delatus est Wintoniam secundum eius desiderium*];[37] and, lastly, a paralysed man who decided to go to Saint Swithin's tomb, planned to be carried there in a litter.[38]

In all these examples the descriptions could be taken to indicate the passivity of the impaired individuals, yet the reader is informed of their directing their own care. How many other people who were carried in litters, taken, brought, or led to saints and shrines - on the surface demonstrating passivity – were really the force

---

[24] 'Miracula S. Swithuni' 2003, 672.
[25] Ælfric 1966, 66.
[26] Bede (1969b: 258).
[27] Anonymous (2003b: 656).
[28] Bede (1969a: 34).
[29] Lantfred of Winchester (2003: 290).
[30] Lantfred of Winchester (2003: 29); Wulfstan of Winchester (2003: 486).
[31] Wulfstan of Winchester (2003: 480); Anonymous (2003b: 660).
[32] Wulfstan of Winchester (2003: 480); Anonymous (2003b: 660).
[33] Ælfric of Eynsham (1881: 162).
[34] Lantfred of Winchester 2003, 291.
[35] Lantfred of Winchester 2003, 279, repeated Wulfstan of Winchester 2003, 471.
[36] 'Miracula S. Swithuni' 2003, 675.
[37] Lantfred of Winchester 2003, 297.
[38] Ælfric 1966, 69.

behind those actions - demonstrating agency? This should stand as a reminder to historians not to accept descriptions of impaired people at face value and consider generic and lexical conventions.

Other examples of a lack of agency seem to have been influenced by unrelated factors. Lantfred included a strange passing remark, inserted into another impaired person's miracle story. Upon arriving at Swithun's tomb, the miracle seeker found there 'a little blind woman' [*mulierculam caecutientem*] whom he was instructed by Swithun to remove from the premises.[39] We are told nothing about her or what became of her, apart from the fact that she was denied even the act available to the most desperate and desolate – prayer for God's mercy and intervention. What led the author to describe such a lack of agency? Was it her gender? Was she socially inferior, expressed by the diminutive? Lantfred does not provide an answer. It remains a tantalizing glimpse into the play of social factors beyond impairment in constructions of agency. There are other, less stark but more informative, examples of subordination in the sources.

A hunchbacked man was cared for by his employer and followed his suggestion that he seek a miracle at Saint Swithun's tomb,[40] while at Abbess Aelfflaed's monastery a nun who suffered from a chronic pain in the head was cured after the abbess wrapped her head with a miraculous girdle sent to her by Saint Cuthbert,[41] and a nun with a withered hand begged her abbess for permission to use Saint Oswald's relics.[42] In these examples, subordinate status – to an employer or an abbess – diminished the impaired person's agency. Children were often (though not always) passive in their care and cure narratives.[43]

A more complex example is that of Wulfwig, a 'rustic' [*rusticorum*] who went blind, did not receive his own vision regarding his condition (as was often the case in the sources, and in *The Life of King Edward the Confessor* in particular), but was rather instructed by 'a citizen's wife' [*materfamilias*] how he should seek healing after she had a vision about him.[44] This is a rare example of an impaired person's cure being revealed in a vision to someone other than him- or herself. The fact that Wulfwig did not only not make choices regarding his care but was not even seen fit by the author to receive his own vision, suggests that a very great level of passivity

---

[39] Lantfred of Winchester 2003, 281.
[40] Ibid, 689.
[41] Bede 1969b, 233.
[42] Byrhtfrth 2009, 145.
[43] Wulfstan of Winchester 2003, 395-397, 468, 483; 'Miracula S. Swithuni' 2003, 653, 659, 657; Alcuin 1982, 35; Bede 1969a, 59, 65; Bede 1969b, 259; Anonymous Monk of Lindisfarne 1969, 119; Wulfstan of Winchester 1991, 67, 69.
[44] The Life King Edward Who Rests at Westminster 1992, 98-99.

was expected by the author, and perhaps by the audience. This could have resulted from his status, as in the above examples. Such examples of passivity should not necessarily be understood as influenced by physical conditions and might simply be cases of social hierarchies. The fact that several of the sources containing these examples also have ones of the agency of impaired people, could support such an interpretation.

However, at times, a person's lack of agency was at odds with his or her social status. Notably, that was the case with Bonifacius, a noble man from Ravenna, who 'became suddenly dumb, [færlice dumb], and was healed after his wife requested a visit from Saint Apollinaris.'[45] Considering that other mute people were active in their care and cure narratives, this lack of agency is telling. While wives and husbands were equally expected to care for an ailing spouse (about a tenth of specified caregivers in the sources are spouses), this is a unique example of the passivity of an impaired man to the level of a transference of agency to his wife. This might be explained by the fact that this episode was part of a retelling of the life of Apollinaris and did not originate in Anglo-Saxon England. Ælfric may have simply repeated the details of an established story, without making a point about Bonifacius' agency. However, as Ælfric made calculated decisions regarding which miracle stories to repeat in his texts, he might have been more conscious of the resulting impression.

The only other example in this vein is found in the *Life of Swithun*. In Wulfstan of Winchester, a paralysed noble man relayed to his wife an elaborate vision he had, and she suggested he go to Saint Swithun's tomb to seek a cure. Her advice 'please[d]' [*placuit*] the man and he acted accordingly.[46] The *Miracula S. Swithuni* emphasised the wife's role even more, having her not only suggest an interpretation of the vision, but declare its meaning.[47] In these examples, although it is the wife who suggests the pilgrimage, much of the initiative remains with the husband: he is the one to have the vision, and his approval is needed for the pilgrimage to take place. While Bonifacius is an example of a total loss of agency, the paralysed man from the *Life of Swithun* is a more ambiguous case. These two examples are the only extant ones of a lack of agency in care and cure, without the mitigating circumstances of subordinate social status or lexical conventions. Above all, they stand as a reminder that no society, and no source, had monolithic cultural perceptions.

---

[45] Ælfric 1881, 476-477.
[46] Lantfred of Winchester 2003, 329; Wulfstan of Winchester 2003, 545.
[47] 'Miracula S. Swithuni' 2003, 675.

The fluidity of agency in care and cure

The agency of impaired people was not always fixed. One story from the *Life of Swithun* illustrated how is could change according to circumstances. Æthelsige, a cleric who had a 'great hump' [*ingentem gibbum*], had a vision of a 'highly-skilled physician' [*medicum... peritissimum*] in Winchester. He immediately left the monastery where he was raised (against the wishes of the monks who raised him), and set out for Winchester, and was taken in by a local moneyer with whom he lived for six-months. Up to this point, Æthelsige had exhibited high levels of agency - receiving a vision, interpreting it, defying the wishes of the monks in his monastery, and leaving on a pilgrimage. However, once he entered into an arrangement of unofficial charity with the moneyer, his agency was drastically reduced. During that period, he was described in passive language, called the moneyer '*mi pater*', followed his instructions, and was taken by him to various places, as it pleased the moneyer.[48] It seems that much like above examples, as the circumstances emphasised Æthelsige's subordinate social position his agency was curtailed.

The story closes with a negotiation of agency: after living in Winchester for six months, Æthelsige had a second vision. This time, he did not act upon it independently, but reported the vision to the moneyer, who then instructed him to return to sleep, saying that in the morning he will take Æthelsige to Saint Swithun's tomb. In the morning, the moneyer suggested a course of action and sought Æthelsige's agreement.[49] On the one hand, Æthelsige could still receive a vision, and his opinion was still solicited. On the other, he had lost the initiative he had originally displayed. However, the audience was not left with a final view of Æthelsige as without agency. While the monks at Winchester erroneously decided the he was cured thanks to the intercession of Saint Martin, Æthelsige insisted that it had been Swithun who had cured him, which, Lantfred assures us, had been the correct interpretation.[50]

Conclusion

I have shown how Anglo-Saxon sources accepted and encouraged the view that impaired people should have control over their care and cure processes. Secular and religious, men and women, young and old, were able to exercise their agency, as evident in their social interactions (instructing and commanding others in

---

[48] Lantfred of Winchester 2003, 267-273; Wulfstan of Winchester 2003, 423.
[49] Lantfred of Winchester 2003, 267-273; Wulfstan of Winchester 2003, 423.
[50] Lantfred of Winchester 2003, 273-275.

how to assist and care for them), in their actions (described in active language), in their decision making (at times going against possible authority figures, and able to decide on a course of action without criticism - even when wrong), and their conceptualisation (as having mental faculties, as able to explain their own impairment, as exercising authority).

An analysis of examples of a lack of agency reveals how factors other than impairment influenced it. Complete agency was not always available to impaired people and reliance on physical help was an important factor in their lived experiences. Social status also played a part: subordination, social liminality, or even conditions of patronage, all brought with them diminished agency to impaired individuals. The subordination of impairment to other social factors strengthens my conclusion that, often, impairment was not seen as an important element in constructions of agency.

While to a modern reader generic conventions (which presented miracle recipients primarily as bodies on which saints act) and physical dependence (which largely characterised the lived realities of impaired people) can create an impression of a great passivity, the sources in fact emphasised the 'still sound' minds of impaired people, and their agency. To frame the question in the context of Disability Studies - was impairment constructed as disabling agency and control of one's own fate? In Anglo-Saxon narrative sources, the answer is - no. And to a large extent, that was the result of emphasizing mental ability over physical disability.

Bibliography

Ælfric 1992. St Swithun, Bishop, in G. I. Needham (ed.), *Lives of Three English Saints*: 60–81. Exeter: University of Exeter Press.

Ælfric 1881. *Aelfric's Lives of Saints: Being a Set of Sermons on Saint's Days Formerly Observed by the English Church*. Trans. and ed. W. W. Skeat. London: Early English Text Society.

Æthelwulf 1967. *De Abbatibus*. Trans. and ed. A. Campbell. Oxford: Oxford University Press.

Alcuin 1982. *The Bishops and Saints of York*. Trans. and ed. P. Goodman. Oxford: Oxford University Press.

Aldhelm 2009. The *Carmen de Virginitate*, in M. Lapidge and J. Rosier (trans and eds), *Aldhelm: The Poetic Works*: 102–167. Cambridge: Brewer.

Anonymous 2003a. Epitome Translationis et Miraculorum S. Swithuni, in M. Lapidge (trans. and ed.), *The Cult of St Swithun*: 563–573. Oxford: Oxford University Press.

Anonymous 2003b. Miracula S. Swithuni, in M. Lapidge (trans. and ed.), *The Cult of St Swithun*: 647–697. Oxford: Oxford University Press.

Anonymous Monk of Lindisfarne 1969. The Life of St Cuthbert by an Anonymous Author, in B. Colgrave (trans. and ed.), *Two Lives of Saint Cuthbert: A Life by an Anonymous Monk of Lindisfarne and Bede's Prose Life,* 59–139. New York: Macmillan.

Barlow, F. (trans. and ed.) 1992. *The Life King Edward Who Rests at Westminster.* Oxford: Oxford University Press.

Bede 1969a. The Life of St Cuthbert by Bede, in B. Colgrave (trans. and ed.), *Two Lives of Saint Cuthbert: A Life by an Anonymous Monk of Lindisfarne and Bede's Prose Life:* 141–307. New York: Macmillan.

Bede 1969b. *Ecclesiastical History of the English People.* Trans. and ed. B. Colgrave and R. A. B. Mynors. Oxford: Oxford University Press.

Bragg. L. 1997. From the Mute God to the Lesser God: Disability in Medieval Celtic and Old Norse Literature. *Disability & Society* 12(2): 165–178.

Byrhtferth of Ramsey 2009. Vita S. Oswaldi, in M. Lapidge (trans. and ed.), *Byrhtferth of Ramsey: The Lives of St Oswald and St Ecgwine*, 1–203. Oxford: Oxford University Press.

Fell, C. E. (ed.) 1971. *Edward King and Martyr.* Leeds: University of Leeds, School of English.

Lantfred of Winchester 2003. Translatio et miracula S. Swithuni, in M. Lapidge (trans. and ed.), *The Cult of St Swithun*: 251–333. Oxford: Oxford University Press.

Lee, C. 2012. Disability, in J. Stodnick and R. Trilling (eds), *A Handbook of Anglo-Saxon Studies*: 23–38. Chichester: John Wiley & Sons.

Reindal, S. M. 1999. Independence, Dependence, Interdependence: Some Reflections on the Subject and Personal Autonomy. *Disability & Society* 14(3): 353–367.

Wilkerson, A. 2002. Disability, Sex Radicalism, and Political Agency. *NWSA Journal* 14(3): 33–57.

Wulfstan of Winchester 2003. Narratio Metrica De S. Swithuno, in M. Lapidge (trans. and ed.), *The Cult of St Swithun,* 371–551. Oxford: Oxford University Press.

Wulfstan of Winchester 1991. *The Life of Æthelwold.* Trans. and eds. M. Lapidge and M. Winterbottom. Oxford: Oxford University Press.

Mobility Limitations and Assistive Aids in the Merovingian Burial Record

Cathrin Hähn

Burials can be a good source for evidence of body-related social differences like gender, age and dis/ability. Concerning approaches to dis/ability in the early Middle Ages,[1] the archaeological sources and especially burials are connected closely with the body itself and therefore to pathological features. Furthermore, burials may include evidence of compensatory objects in cases of physical limitations and impairments. Burials may shed light on living and dealing with limitations, although they may not necessarily represent the everyday life of the deceased, but rather a special ritual arranged by the community. Thus, whether the mobility limitation of a person played a role or not for the community could also become visible in the burial.

At this point, there are not many recorded cases of mobility limitations apart from age-related problems like osteoarthritis. Possible problems in detecting them are similar to the general problems in finding palaeopathological conditions[2]— missing limbs are usually not recorded clearly, especially not in older excavations. Skeletons from older excavations may not have been preserved appropriately, with the delicate bones of fingers or feet being lost or remains of different individuals being mixed up due to external causes, as happened to some skeletal series from southern Germany during World War II.[3] However, bioarchaeological analysis is essential and ideally carried out during the excavation. In the case of an amputation, it is sometimes not easy to determine whether a limb has been removed during life or peri-/postmortem.[4] The latter case would not necessarily suggest any kind of mobility impairment of an individual during his or her lifetime.

---

[1] For example, Metzler (2006), Lee (2011), Crawford and Lee (2010), Crawford and Lee (2014).
[2] Simone Kahlow recorded possible restrictions in tracing archaeological evidence for prostheses and artificial body parts in Kahlow (2009: 203).
[3] This concerns the first 344 skeletons of a total of 630 burials from the skeletal series of Schretzheim, Baden-Württemberg: Koch (1977: 8) (the excavation of the burial field is probably not complete), and a greater part of the series of Mengen, Baden-Württemberg: Walter (2008: 20).
[4] Roberts (2000: 344).

Prostheses or other assistive aids, like those discovered in the burial complexes presented below, are therefore to be viewed as outstandingly valuable pieces of evidence. These objects are illustrative of the kind of compensation that has been undertaken and indicate that the affected person would likely have lived with a missing limb and a possible impairment for a significant amount of time. Reasons for the loss of a limb or other body parts are, again, difficult to establish with any certainty. One problem is that in most cases only the healthy part is found in archaeological contexts. Finds of removed parts of limbs could reveal pathology, but such finds are rather unlikely to be made, as there are no specific sites where human body parts are known to have been buried or disposed. One could imagine cemeteries for this purpose, but in fact, there are very few examples. An exception is one case from the early medieval cemetery of Herrenberg, Baden-Württemberg, Germany, where a hand, probably cut off during a fight, was kept in a small wooden box and buried sometime after the separation together with the individual's body. The stump on the arm showed advanced signs of healing, suggesting that the person survived the amputation for at least several months.[5]

Another possible reason for lost limbs in the archaeological evidence would be amputation in the context of corporeal punishment.[6] As already shown, several circumstances could lead to an amputation: from legal punishment or violent injury to medical amputation due to an accident, burn injuries or freezing. One of the few cases in which the reasons for an amputation are obvious is an amputated foot from early modern Lübeck in Schleswig-Holstein, Germany, which bears some discoloration on the toes that might be the result of an infection of the soft tissue that ultimately led to the amputation.[7] The reasons for the amputation might be irrelevant for the bioarchaeological feature, but for the social life of the affected person, they could have been crucial: while those who had an amputation in the context of corporeal punishment were intentionally stigmatised, others with similar visible bodily differences could have a document drawn up confirming that they sustained the loss of a body part in another way than by legal prosecution.[8]

Mobility Aids: Production, Spectrum and Preservation

The wide spectrum of possible types of assistive aids for compensation or help with mobility limitations during the early Middle Ages calls for great sensitivity in recognising the varying remains of these aids during the excavation, as well as

---

[5] Wahl (2007: 95–96).
[6] Buckberry (2014: 144–148); Hähn (2017).
[7] Herrmann (1984: 83); Kahlow (2012: 559–560).
[8] Timmer, Schuster, and Nolte (2017).

in the subsequent interpretation of the finds in context. Especially when a limb is missing, attention should be paid to the possibility of an assistive aid being situated in the place of utilisation (i.e., instead of a missing lower leg), but also elsewhere in the grave. With the re-examination of older material, particularly nonidentified objects from preserved burial assemblages, more evidence of the use of assistive aids could be found, especially among the great number of burials from the Merovingian period.

The presented cases allow some conclusions about the people who built those assistive aids: Almost certainly there were individual craftsmen who had the knowledge and skill necessary for building prostheses, ortheses and other assistive aids. The few objects currently recorded are most likely not the only ones that would have been in use at that time in history. The actual extent of use of 'specially designed, "tailor-made"' mobility aids must lie between this observation on the basis of archaeological finds and Irina Metzler's conclusion that they were not accessible to all who would have needed them.[9] Maybe there were specialised smiths or carpenters who manufactured such products, as they were often constructed from different materials such as wood, metal and leather, combined to form a single object, which requires knowledge to deal with several different materials. A separate trade like that of today's orthopaedic technician, however, presumably did not exist during the Middle Ages.[10]

Redesigned everyday objects, which Metzler sees as the most common design for medieval mobility aids,[11] would possibly not be preserved when made of wood, or not recognised in their function when found in early medieval burials. However, another factor could limit the number and possibility of finding traces of assistive aids: burial customs themselves, especially the custom of furnishing the dead with material goods. In this context, the possibility of not endowing the dead with modified everyday items is also imaginable, because of a relative 'ignobility' or lack of individuality—which, in contrast, specially manufactured and professional mobility aids could have. So, a presumably prevalent use of assistive aids does not lead to an endowment at any given time because, if there were, many more exemplars would have been recorded. The very small number of these assistive aids in burials seems to result from chronologically different habits of including them in the range of common burial offerings. During the 7th century AD, changes in the Merovingian burial customs, which are commonly associated with the increasing influence of Christianity, become apparent. The

---

[9] Metzler (2006: 176).
[10] First master's examination regulations in Germany were established in 1883; Bieringer (2006: 19–20).
[11] Metzler (2006: 176).

most considerable trend of that time becomes manifest in a decrease in the wealth and number of furnished burials. Sebastian Brather detects a serious remodelling of burial customs here: formerly, the contents of graves represented 'collections of objects'; now, the influence of Christianity takes effect, but rather than of a standardisation to unfurnished burials, the means of representation of an individual's status are donated to church trusts.[12] Burial furnishing customs are at their peak during the first half of the 7th century, and therefore a great amount of burials are well datable due to their diverse grave goods. Probably linked with this transition and peaking in the furnishing customs are the cases of furnished assistive aids as well. After that peak, the burial furnishings decrease until the 8th century and the transfer of the burial places to churchyards, and—although the exact reasons for that development are not yet fully formed—a concrete ban of grave goods by the Catholic Church was non-existent, and furnished burials were still common among clerical and secular authorities.[13]

History

A historical (non)transmission of mobility limitations shows how anthropological finds can shed new light on a historical person. Queen Aregond lived about AD 520–565 and was the second wife of the Frankish King Clothaire I. She was buried in the vault of St Dénis near Paris, where her remains were uncovered in 1959 and identified by means of a signet ring with her name on it.[14] The anthropological examination of the skeleton revealed that she had been afflicted with an infection of poliomyelitis or infantile paralysis in childhood, which resulted in the shortening of her left leg because of bone malformations on her left ankle. Her right foot and leg were also affected, but not to the same extent as the left side. This condition must have resulted in at least slight limping.[15] Since poliomyelitis is only dangerous during childhood in phases of bone growth, we can assume that she must have carried the resulting malformations for most of her life and even before she met and married her husband, King Clothaire. Historical sources, however, do not tell us about any physical differences. We are only informed that Aregond became the mother of Chlothaire's son and heir to the throne, Chilperic I of Neustria. It is not known if Aregond was impaired due to those differences or if they hindered her from fulfilling any of her duties, especially considering her social and political background as a member of a noble family and in the role of a queen. Aregond's

---

[12] Brather (2008: 165).
[13] Reindel (1995, 142).
[14] France-Lanord and Fleury (1962: 358–359).
[15] Périn *et al.* (2007, 153).

standing in society demonstrates that bodily differences were not necessarily social obstacles at the time and that there may have been other factors such as noble origin to compensate for impairments. A physically 'imperfect' queen and future mother to the heir was obviously not an impossibility.

Examples of mobility aids

Assistive aids were found in several graves from the 7th to the 9th centuries AD. They were presumably buried with their former user and in those cases were apparently part of an otherwise common assemblage of burial furnishings made up of clothes, jewellery and weapons.

A lower leg orthosis has been discovered in an undisturbed, end-of-7th-century AD burial from Markt Einersheim in Bavaria, Germany.[16] Other items found in this grave include a simple belt buckle, a small knife, a bodkin and the remains of a comb. Furthermore, there was a single spur found next to the right foot. It seems likely that it was only to be worn on the healthy foot, keeping in mind that, at the time in question, *pars-pro-toto* burial objects were not unusual. Examples include assemblages with only one spur (sometimes even carried in a pocket) instead of a pair,[17] as well as others featuring complete pairs. Intriguingly, right below the left foot were the remains of an orthosis: several belts of iron pressed together with organic material sticking to them. The iron belts both had a U-shape and were fitted with leather. Reconstructed, the orthosis would fit below the heel, the iron belts would protect the ankle, and combined with them, a leather inner shoe would probably protect the foot against getting sore. An additional leather band was mounted around the Achilles tendon to prevent the foot from slipping out of the construction.[18] Unfortunately, the bones are preserved so badly that the physiological reason for wearing the orthosis could not be detected. What could be established is merely the estimated age of the deceased man as mature (40 to 60 years). The ends of the long bones are corroded, but on the bones of the right leg, distinct marks of muscle attachment of the lower-leg musculature, which could be caused by straining the healthy leg while sparing the left one, are detectable.[19]

The function of the orthosis surely was to protect the tendons of the ankle after they became weakened due to an earlier trauma. The possible applications of an orthosis are numerous, so it is notable that this is the first recorded case of an

---

[16] Herbold, Pütz, Trentzsch, and Oberpriller (2013).
[17] Herbold *et al.* (2013: 409); Rettner (1997).
[18] Herbold *et al.* (2013: 412–13).
[19] Herbold *et al.* (2013: 412).

early medieval orthosis.[20] The elaborate construction may be seen as proof that the technology was well established, even though relevant objects would not habitually be buried with the user. This shows one of the general problems with burials as archaeological sources: they do not reflect every bodily aspect of everyday life. Instead, the items that go into the burial are filtered by the community, which ultimately selects the grave goods.

A further, and probably better known, example of assistive aids is that of a prosthesis discovered in a late 7th- to early 8th-century AD burial from Griesheim near Darmstadt in Hessia, Germany.[21] The grave was disturbed soon after the burial, mainly in the areas of the head and pelvis. The legs were left in situ, of which the left one was extant only from pelvis to knee. On close inspection, a shell of bronze sheet was found near the left foot. It must be interpreted as the remainder of an otherwise wooden prosthesis. The lower leg had been skilfully exarticulated at the knee joint, but the reason for this (most likely medical) intervention cannot be reconstructed based on the rest of the skeletal remains.[22]

A second type of prosthesis was found in a Swiss cemetery of mostly Romanesque burials from Bonaduz, Bot Valbeuna, Canton Graubünden, Switzerland. It is of the same time as the aforementioned case but differs in its use.[23] The design was intended to protect the stump—it would not have been possible to walk on this exemplar. It was made of a leather bag filled with a pillow of moss and hay, which was reinforced with an iron skid running across. The find, however, did not include fixtures that could have been used to attach the prosthetic to the body, perhaps due to the materials' organic quality. Such a prosthesis may have been used in the hope to facilitate the healing process of the bones. The foot was exarticulated at the ankle joint, but the person (whose sex could not be determined) probably suffered from an inflammatory process that must have been very painful and was possibly accompanied by fever episodes. Small openings for the leaking of pus are visible on the end of the fibula and tibia, where the stump, and therefore the contact area of leg and prosthesis, was situated. The two lower leg bones became fused by bone neoplasm, which is also a sign of infectious processes. The infection did not heal before the death of the person, which presumably occurred no more than one or two years after the amputation.[24]

A very special case, also associated with the field of orthopaedic supplies, comes from the cemetery of Pleidelsheim, Baden-Württemberg, Germany. A young

---

[20] Herbold *et al.* (2013: 413).
[21] Keil (1980); Wahl, Wittwer-Backofen, and Kunter (1997: 347–348).
[22] Keil (1980: 202–203).
[23] Czarnetzki, Uhlig, and Wolf (1983: 93–94).
[24] Czarnetzki, Uhlig, and Wolf (1983: 93).

woman, who died at the age of 18–20 years, was buried here between the years AD 530 and 555.[25] Her foot bones are missing on both sides, and the fibulae and tibiae appear slightly atrophied. The exact reason for the absence of feet is not detectable, as no signs of amputation could be found. Poliomyelitis has been discussed in previous research,[26] but seems implausible as the cause for the loss of both feet. In contrast to the cases presented above, no signs of prostheses, or at least not of a non-organic material, were found below her legs. Nevertheless, situated to the woman's right, within the large wooden burial chamber, are two small boot-shaped vessels made of ceramic. The boots' upper part is designed as biconical pots, the typical contemporary burial vessels in southwestern Germany, whereas the tip is shaped as Poulaines with grooved ornaments. Inside the hollow, remains of organic materials such as moss were found. Moreover, two clamps of bronze found beside the vessels could have been used to attach them to the fabric of an individual's clothing, for instance. Traces of a nonspecified (in the publication) organic material about four millimetres thick was still adhering to the clamps.[27] What is special about the vessels is the paragenesis with the anthropological record of missing foot bones. However, they could almost certainly not have been used for walking on them. If they were used as prostheses, it would likely have been for cosmetic purposes. One could imagine the user sitting with the stumped legs placed in the vessels, which could have been attached to the wearer's trousers by using the clamps. This interpretation is also supported by the fact that the shoes are very small, only 13 centimetres in length. This would correlate with the shoe size of a two-year-old child today. However, the actual utility of the artefact is not clear. This curious find also raises the question why no prostheses made of more practically useful material, such as wood, that the buried individuals might have owned, were buried with them. Such prostheses were not even found elsewhere, e.g., in a non-burial context. Another shoe vessel from the same period was found in Mainz-Hechtsheim, Rheinland-Pfalz, Germany,[28] where it had been placed below the feet of a woman of about 40 years, together with some non-analysed organic grave goods. A third object, from Bronze Age Glauberg, Hessia, Germany, shows that the custom of placing shoe vessels into graves significantly predates the above finds.[29] Nevertheless, the vessels from Pleidelsheim are almost unique finds in that such objects are not always necessarily associated with a special anthropological record. Furthermore, the finds of the bronze clamps provide strong evidence for

---

[25] Koch (2001: 472–474); Wahl *et al.* (1997: 344).
[26] Wahl *et al.* (1997: 344).
[27] Koch (2001: 472–473).
[28] Koch (2011: 218, table 12); Zeller (1996: 679, fig. 549).
[29] Baitinger (2007).

the interpretation as prosthetic means, since no other shoe vessels found up to now carried similar provisions.

Another type of object that must be mentioned in the context of mobility limitations is the so-called *Stabdorne*. They are the foot caps of wooden canes, reinforced with a pin, and, so far, are construed as belonging to weaponry and pilgrims' or bishops' croziers.[30] A few examples are classified as a type of crutches. This designation, of *Stabdorne,* is the most neutral form concerning the wider discussion about their possible function and meaning as burial objects.[31] The majority are dated to somewhere between the 7th and 9th centuries AD and are found in burial contexts. However, a small number have been discovered on settlement sites.[32] For instance, in a burial from St Mary's church in Schleitheim, Switzerland,[33] a woman with all her joints afflicted by arthritic changes would likely have used the walking aid, reinforced with a *Stabdorn*, in her daily life. Canes are also known from medieval pictorial sources,[34] but they may simply represent tools and aids for a variety of purposes, so that many different reconstructions of the entire object, which the *Stabdorn* is part of, seem to be possible. Therefore, the existence of a *Stabdorn* in a burial does not automatically lead to a certain conclusion on the degree of a person's mobility or impairment thereof. Apart from that, age-related mobility impairments are to be interpreted differently (as in unsteadiness) than those caused by accidents, illnesses or violent injury of younger individuals.

Conclusion

These few examples from the early Middle Ages show that manually crafted assistive aids must be considered as being used with more regularity than we could suspect from their sporadic appearance in burial sites. The objects are designed so efficiently and successfully that it would be hard to imagine that they are singular items. The custom of placing a used prosthesis or other aid in the grave with the deceased may only have begun with the general change of burial customs during the 7th century AD. However, the aids cannot be seen as part of a new range of grave goods, as they are more closely associated with the body and seem similar to personal items such as clothes.

---

[30] Steuer (2005: 414–415).
[31] Steuer (2005).
[32] One exemplar comes from the early medieval settlement Heiligenberg near Heidelberg; this case and a brief summary of the discussion in Gross (2012: 451).
[33] Bänteli and Ruckstuhl (1986).
[34] Kühnel (1985: fig. 121).

To verify this thesis, further investigations are required, both of new excavation sites as well as into previously discovered and recorded burials. A fresh look at existing material might increase the number of finds of assistive aids, especially keeping in mind that a good portion of medieval mobility aids could be modified everyday objects.[35]

The growing influence of Christianity and the discourse on the completion of the body on judgement day might be associated with the incorporation of mobility aids after a cultural shift. Those associated items are part of a range of both personal and general items furnishing a grave.[36] In that context, a body could also be completed with the already-in-use prosthesis. Is the allocation of the artificial limb understandable as a proposal to God for including this already 'worldly' adapted body part in the resurrected body? On the one hand, maybe the original limb had not been preserved, and it was hoped that a prosthesis might count as a substitute. On the other hand, we might simply be faced with a consequence of the fact that these aids might not have had any significant value to anyone but the individuals they had been made to fit. In contrast to many other objects in the grave, mobility aids and prostheses could therefore be seen as 'disposed of' appropriately. None of the objects discussed above were physically needed after the death of the individual, not even for laying out of the body during the burial rites. But noting the psychosocial connotation of prostheses, they may have been an important part of one's body in making it intact again. Wholeness might have mattered. Therefore, including such objects in the grave might be a psychologically significant act.

In the context of dis/ability, a change of the body image that also manifests in burial rites is unmistakable when the influence of Christianity increases. Like other *rites de passage*,[37] burials must have produced, renewed and transformed body images, especially those burial rites of the early Middle Ages in which the body was decorated and equipped for the afterworld and laid out to be visible for at least parts of the public. If we take burial rites as a possible occasion for the demonstration of social status, concurrent transporting and renegotiating body images is almost unpreventable, for the body is the most important requisite in this event. In the context of dis/ability, these changes in body image could reflect on issues like health and sickness. Aregond and the contemporaneous burial of the young woman from Pleidelsheim are early examples of individuals with mobility limitations, and in contrast to later evidence, no clear sign of a perceived impairment could be found in the burial furnishings. The offside position of the

---

[35] Metzler (2006: 176).
[36] Schmitz-Esser (2014: 19–25); Metzler (2006: 55–62).
[37] Van Gennep (1986).

shoe vessels in the Pleidelsheim burial shows that they did not belong (or no longer belonged) to the body itself—at least at the time of the interment.

Mobility aids as a type of grave goods are not only highly interesting in themselves but also, and especially, in relation to many other issues such as questions of gender and age. As the latest finds from Markt Einersheim, Bavaria, have illustrated, closer investigations of burial sites would certainly generate more data relevant to a better understanding of the significance of mobility aids and dis/ability in the early Middle Ages.

Bibliography

Baitinger, H. 2007. Ein Schuhgefäß der Urnenfelderzeit vom Glauberg, Wetteraukreis (Hessen). *Germania* 85: 47–59.

Bänteli, K. and Ruckstuhl, B. 1986. Die Stiftergräber der Kirche St. Maria zu Schleitheim. *Archäologie der Schweiz/Archéologie suisse/Archeologia svizzera* 9: 68–79.

Bieringer, S. 2006. Orthopädie-Technik, in W. Knoche (ed.), *Prothesen der unteren Extremität. Die Entwicklung vom Altertum bis 1930*: 8–23. Dortmund: Bundesfachschule für Orthopädietechnik.

Brather, S. 2008. Bestattungsrituale zur Merowingerzeit: Frühmittelalterliche Reihengräber und der Umgang mit dem Tod, in C. Kümmel, B. Schweizer and U. Veit (eds), *Körperinszenierung—Objektsammlung—Monumentalisierung. Totenritual und Grabkult in frühen Gesellschaften*, Tübinger Archäologische Taschenbücher 6: 151–180. Münster: Waxmann.

Buckberry, J. 2014. Osteological evidence of corporal and capital punishment in later Anglo-Saxon England, in J. P. Gates and N. Marafioti (eds), *Capital and Corporal Punishment in Anglo-Saxon England*, Anglo-Saxon Studies 23: 131–148. Woodbridge: Boydell & Brewer.

Crawford, S. and Lee, C. (eds) 2010. *Bodies of Knowledge: Cultural Interpretations of Illness and Medicine in Medieval Europe*, Studies in Early Medicine 1. Oxford: Archaeopress.

Crawford, S. and Lee, C. (eds) 2014. *Social Dimensions of Medieval Disease and Disability*, Studies in Early Medicine 3. Oxford: Archaeopress.

Czarnetzki, A., Uhlig, C., and Wolf, R. 1983. *Skelette erzählen. Menschen des frühen Mittelalters im Spiegel der Anthropologie und Medizin*, 2nd ed. Stuttgart: Württembergisches Landesmuseum.

France-Lanord, M. and Fleury, M. 1962. Das Grab der Arnegundis in Saint-Denis. *Germania*, 40: 341–359.

Gross, U. 2012. Die mittelalterlichen und neuzeitlichen Keramik-, Metall- und Beinfunde, in U. Gross, P. Marzloff, and F. Klein (eds), *Forschungen zum Heiligenberg* bei Heidelberg: Forschungsgeschichte, Fundmaterial, Restaurierung, Forschungen und Berichte der Archäologie des Mittelalters in Baden-Württemberg, 32: 393–563. Stuttgart: Theiss.

Hähn, C. 2017. Körperstrafen im archäologischen Befund, in C. Nolte, B. Frohne, U. Halle, and S. Kerth (eds), *Dis/ability History der Vormoderne. Ein Handbuch / Premodern Dis/ability History. A Companion*: 307-314. Affalterbach: Didymos.

Herbold, B., Pütz, A., Trentzsch, H., and Oberpriller, C. 2013. Hilfe für einen Fusslahmen. Zum Befund einer Fussschiene des Frühen Mittelalters aus Markt Einersheim (Lkr. Kitzingen), *Archäologisches Korrespondenzblatt* 43(3): 409–422.

Herrmann, B. 1984. Ein amputierter Fuss aus der frühneuzeitlichen Kloake der Lübecker Fronerei. *Lübecker Schriften zur Archäologie und Kulturgeschichte* 8: 81–84.

Kahlow, S. 2009. Prothesen im Mittelalter: ein Überblick aus archäologischer Sicht, in C. Nolte (ed.), *Homo Debilis: Behinderte—Kranke—Versehrte in der Gesellschaft des Mittelalters*: 203–224. Korb: Didymos.

Kahlow, S. 2012. Zur Frage des archäologischen Nachweises scharfrichterlicher Medizin. Eine Miszelle, in J. Auler (ed.), *Richtstättenarchäologie* 3:556–562. Dormagen: archaeotopos.

Keil, B. 1980. Eine Prothese aus einem fränkischen Grab von Griesheim, Kreis Darmstadt-Dieburg. *Fundberichte aus Hessen* 17-18: 195-211.

Koch, U. 1977. *Das Reihengräberfeld bei Schretzheim*, Vol. 2. Berlin: Mann.

Koch, U. 2001. *Das alamannisch-fränkische Gräberfeld bei Pleidelsheim,* Forschungen und Berichte zur Vor- und Frühgeschichte in Baden-Württemberg 60. Stuttgart: Theiss.

Koch, U. 2011. *Das frühmittelalterliche Gräberfeld von Mainz-Hechtsheim*, Mainzer Archäologische Schriften Vol. 11. Mainz: Generaldirektion Kulturelles Erbe Rheinland-Pfalz.

Kühnel, H. 1985. *Alltag im Spätmittelalter*. Graz: Styria (Edition Kaleidoskop).

Lee, C. 2011. Disease, in H. Hamerow, D. A. Hinton, and S. Crawford (eds) *The Oxford Handbook of Anglo-Saxon Archaeology*: 704–726. Oxford: Oxford University Press.

Metzler, I. 2006. *Disability in Medieval Europe: Thinking About Physical Impairment During the High Middle Ages, c. 1100–1400*. London: Routledge.

Périn, P., Calligaro, T., Buchet, L., Cassiman, L. L., Darton, Y. et al. 2007. Neue Erkenntnisse zum Arnegundegrab. Ergebnisse der Metallanalysen und der Untersuchungen organischer Überreste aus Sarkophag 49 der Basilika von Saint-Denis. *Acta Praehistorica et Archaeologica* 39: 147–179.

Reindel, K. 1995. Grabbeigaben und die Kirche. *Zeitschrift für bayerische Landesgeschichte* 58: 141–145.

Rettner, A. 1997. Sporen der Älteren Merowingerzeit. *Germania* 75(1): 133–157.

Roberts, C. A. 2000. Trauma in biocultural perspective: past, present and future work in Britain, in M. Cox and S. Mays (eds), *Human Osteology: In Archaeology and Forensic Science*: 337–356. London: Greenwich Medical Media.

Schmitz-Esser, R. 2014. *Der Leichnam im Mittelalter. Einbalsamierung, Verbrennung und die kulturelle Konstruktion des toten Körpers*, Mittelalter-Forschungen 48. Ostfildern: Jan Thorbecke.

Steuer, H. 2005. s.v. Stab § 5. Archäologisch, in H. Beck, D. Geuenich, and H. Steuer (eds), *Reallexikon der Germanischen Altertumskunde 29 (Skírnismál—Stiklestad)*: 414–418. Berlin: De Gruyter.

Timmer, S., Schuster, P. and Nolte, C. 2017, Leibesstrafen im Spätmittelalter: Rechtsverordnungen und Rechtspraxis, in C. Nolte, B. Frohne, U. Halle, and S. Kerth (eds), *Dis/ability History der Vormoderne. Ein Handbuch / Premodern Dis/ability History. A Companion*: 316-317. Affalterbach: Didymos.

Van Gennep, A. 1986. *Übergangsriten (Les rites de passage)*. Frankfurt: Campus.

Wahl, J. 2007. *Karies, Kampf & Schädelkult*, Materialhefte zur Archäologie 79. Stuttgart: Theiss.

Wahl, J., Wittwer-Backofen, U., and Kunter, M. 1997. Zwischen Masse und Klasse: Alamannen im Blickfeld der Anthropologie, in K. Fuchs (ed.), *Die Alamannen—Ausstellungskatalog*: 337–348. Stuttgart: Theiss.

Walter, S. 2008. Das frühmittelalterliche Gräberfeld von Mengen (Kr. Breisgau-Hochschwarzwald), unpublished DPhil thesis, Ludwig-Maximilians-Universität Munich, viewed 29 July 2017, <https://edoc.ub.uni-muenchen.de/9450/1/Walter_Susanne_G.pdf>.

Wamers, E. and Périn, P. (eds) 2012. *Königinnen der Merowinger. Adelsgräber aus den Kirchen von Köln, Saint-Denis, Chelles und Frankfurt am Main*. Regensburg: Schnell + Steiner.

Zeller, G. 1996. Tracht der Frauen, in K. von Welck, A. Wieczorek, and H. Ament (eds), *Die Franken. Wegbereiter Europas. Vor 1500 Jahren: König Chlodwig und seine Erben*. Mainz: Philipp von Zabern.

Tearing the Face in Grief and Rape: Cheek Rending in Medieval Iberia, *c.* 1100–1300

Rachel Welsh

> E a entrante la vila ond' ele natura era,
> meteu mui fort' apelido e ouve o rostro rascado ...
> E meteu mui grandes vozes e disse que a forçara
>
> At the entrance to his home town,
> she began to cry out loudly and scratched her face.
> She gave great shouts and said that the youth had forced her ...[1]
>
> Cantiga 355, *Cantigas de Santa María*

Cantiga 355 of the *Cantigas de Santa Maria,* a collection of lyric poems composed or commissioned by King Alfonso X of Castile between 1257 and 1283, tells the story of a young woman who, having been rejected by a prospective lover, took revenge by falsely accusing him of rape. The woman performed the customary gestures of a victim of rape—she appeared in the town *rostro rascado,* with a scratched face. The man was subsequently convicted and sentenced to execution, his escape from the hangman's noose effected only through the miraculous intervention of the Virgin Mary.[2] Although the woman's tearing of her face appears only as a side note in this story, detailing how she lodged her false claim of rape, it sheds light on the standard processes for rape accusations in medieval Castile and León during the 12th and 13th centuries. Rather than testifying verbally or providing character witness to swear on her behalf, as with other types of crimes, the raped woman physically demonstrated the validity of her claim by tearing her face, rending her cheeks until they bled.

Cheek rending was also part of the standard repertoire of ritual mourning practices in medieval Iberia, and the gesture has typically been understood as an emotional expression, an outward sign of internal despair or grief. We may misunderstand cheek rending, however, if we take it only as an emotional sign.

---

[1] Cantiga 355, in Mettmann (1964: 261), translated in Kulp-Hill (2000: 432–434).
[2] For a more thorough analysis of this *cantiga,* see Scarborough (2012: 241).

Legal sources—particularly the municipal legal codes that proliferated during the 13th century—show that the same gesture of cheek rending could function as both emotional truth and legal truth. The present study examines the practice of cheek rending in medieval Castile and León as a bodily gesture with social, legal and physical significance. First, cheek rending functioned as a social gesture, as women tore their cheeks both in claiming rape and as part of the traditional rituals of mourning, which involved not only crying and vocal laments but also self-injurious physical gestures such as beating the breast and tearing the hair, clothing and face. Second, cheek rending functioned as a gendered gesture with legal implications and meaning; women did not tear their faces merely to reflect the social disgrace or emotional distress of violation, but because the municipal legal codes in many towns specifically required women to rend their cheeks in order to initiate a valid claim of rape. Cheek rending was therefore a legal maneuver, not only an emotional expression. Third, the gesture must also be understood as a physical action with bodily consequences; sculpted, painted or literary figures tore their cheeks in stylised grief, but flesh-and-blood women also clawed at their faces, leaving painful—and perhaps even permanent—marks on real bodies. Cheek rending as a shared gesture connects widows and raped women, but it may also suggest a connection between women's bodies and medieval conceptions of proof and truth.

Cheek Rending as Ritual Mourning

Cheek rending in medieval Iberia was part of a larger constellation of Mediterranean mourning practices reaching back to the classical period. In this traditional funeral ritual, mourners, whether family members or those paid by the family to mourn publicly, uncovered their heads, beat their chests, and clawed at their hair, clothing, and faces, blood streaming from their self-inflicted wounds. This form of ritual mourning appears throughout 12th- and 13th-century sources, often under the umbrella term *llanto,* or lament. As Muñoz Fernández argues, the sounds, words and gestures of grief could function interchangeably to signify the same performance of mourning; people understood that they could 'hacer llanto con la boca, con las manos, y con los ojos', could perform *llanto* with the mouth, the hands and the eyes.[3]

Castilian chronicles during the period abound with references to *llanto* and the mutilating physical gestures of mourning.[4] For example, in the *Chronicon regum legionensium* (c. 1121–1132), Bishop Pelayo of Oviedo recounts the outpouring of

---

[3] Muñoz Fernández (2009: here 138, 118).
[4] On depictions of mourning in chronicles and other narrative sources, see Muñoz Fernández (2009: 110–118).

public grief at the death of King Alfonso VI of León in 1109, observing that 'the counts, knights (both the nobles and those not of noble birth), and citizens tore out their hair and rent their clothes, the women scratched their faces, and they sprinkled ashes and with great moaning and heaviness of heart they shouted to the heavens'.[5] Bishop Pelayo relates most deaths with a simple *mortuus est,* reserving his elaborate descriptions of mourning for the death of Alfonso VI, whom he had known personally and whose burial he likely actually witnessed. His account reflects standard mourning gestures and can be understood as both descriptive and prescriptive. Noble men and women almost certainly lamented and tore themselves in grief at Alfonso's death, and Pelayo uses their extreme mourning to emphasise the king's greatness; these were proper mourning gestures, worthy of a king. The author of the *Chronica Adefonsi Imperatoris,* written in the mid- to late 12th century, appears to have borrowed directly from Bishop Pelayo's account in his description of the death of King Alfonso I of Aragón in 1134: again, 'both nobles and commoners, citizens and foreigners . . .tore out their hair and rent their clothes, and the women scratched their faces'.[6] The *Crónica latina de los reyes de Castilla* (c. 1236) describes a similar scene at the death of the young Infante Fernando of León in 1211: well-born men wore sackcloth and covered their heads with ashes, while virgins tore at their faces.[7] The Romance chronicle *Primera Crónica General* (c. 1282–1284) describes the crowds of mourners at the death of King Fernando III of Castile in 1252 in more emotional terms:

> And who saw so many ladies of high status, and so many maidens walking wild-haired and scratched, tearing their faces and peeling them back in blood and in open wounds? Who saw so many princes, so many rich men, so many nobles, so many knights, so many generous men walking around wailing, crying out, pulling out their hair and tearing their foreheads and doing such great cruelties to themselves?[8]

---

[5] *Chronicon regum legionensium*: 'Tunc comites et milites, nobiles et innobiles, siue et ciues, descaluatis capitibus, scissis uestibus, rupte facies / mulierum, asperso cinere cum magno gemitu et dolore cordis dabant uoces usque ad celos' (Sánchez Alonso 1924: 87–88; translated in Barton and Fletcher 2000: 88–89).

[6] *Chronica Adefonsi Imperatoris*, cap. 61, in Barton and Fletcher (2000: 189).

[7] 'Nusquam luctus aberati, seniores consperserunt capita sua cinere, induti sunt omnes saccis et cilicio, virgines omnes scalide, facies terre penitus inmutata est'. Desamparados Cabanes Pecourt (1964: 41).

[8] '¿Et quién vio tanta duenna de alta guisa et tanta donzella andar descabennadas et rascadas, ronpiendo las fazes et tornandolas en sangre et en carne biva? ¿Quién vio tanto infante, tanto rico omne, tanto infançon, tanto cavallero, tanto omne de prestar andando baladrando, dando bozes, mesando sus cabellos et ronpiendo las fruentes et faziendo en sy

The author seems somewhat taken aback by such high-status mourners tearing their faces, but he depicts this kind of mourning ritual as appropriate and good, a marvel—*maravilla*—that honored Fernando in his death. The chronicle may exaggerate this scene to highlight Fernando's glory as a king, but the embellishment would lie in the numbers and rank of the mourners, not in their actions; individual mourners tore their cheeks for the deaths of relatives, and cities of high-born and wealthy mourners tore their cheeks for the deaths of kings.

Like the chronicle accounts of mourning, the songs and images in the *Cantigas de Santa María* both reflect lived practice and reinforce the centrality of full-bodied and even self-injurious gestures to conceptions of ideal mourning, and women's mourning in particular. The *cantigas* relate numerous miracles in which Mary either heals the grievously wounded or revives the dead. Most of these depict the family's mourning before the miracle; both men and women wail, tear their clothing and pull at their hair, and women rend their cheeks.[9] Furthermore, although a few *cantigas* mention cheek rending explicitly, cheek rending can be assumed as a feature of mourning even in *cantigas* that only describe weeping or *llanto*. For example, one *cantiga* tells the story of a licentious knight who reformed his life after a visitation from the Virgin Mary and died a good death; although the text does not mention mourning, the accompanying miniatures include a deathbed scene, complete with mourners—five figures stand by the bed, and the two women tear their cheeks in grief.[10] While the women themselves do not figure in the larger story of the *cantiga*, the image of them rending their cheeks symbolises the knight's honorable death. In other *cantigas*, the bodily gestures of mourning seem more tied to actual practice and play a role in the narrative plot; in *cantiga* 21, a mother whose miraculously conceived child died of a fever soon after birth 'almost lost her mind over his loss and tore her cheeks in grief'.[11] In another *cantiga* about a child who had died, the poet exclaims: 'I find it painful to tell you how greatly his mother grieved for him then. She cried loudly, tearing her hair, and did not cease twisting the fingers of her hands and clawing at her arms'.[12] These *cantigas* use the visceral horror of the women's self-injurious mourning gestures to underscore the reality of the children's death and their subsequent miraculous resurrection, but

---

fuertes cruezas?' In Menéndez Pidal (1906: cap. 1134, p. 773). My own translation.

[9] The *cantigas* most often tell of mothers grieving for their children, but *cantigas* that mention both parents usually describe them as mourning equally; one *cantiga* even tells of a father who 'smote his cheeks and snatched out his hair and made great mourning' at the death of his only and beloved son. Cantiga 323, Kulp-Hill (2000: 391).

[10] Cantiga 152, Kulp-Hill (2000: 186). Image in El Escorial manuscript of the *cantigas*, miniature reproduced in Dillard (1984: plate 20).

[11] Cantiga 21, Kulp-Hill (2000: 30).

[12] Cantiga 331, Kulp-Hill (2000: 402).

they also show that cheek rending and other physical acts of self-harm were seen as standard mourning practice, especially for women.

In the *Cantigas de Santa María* and in everyday life in 13th-century Castile and León, cheek rending functioned as a public expression of appropriate female grief. While women may indeed have torn their cheeks as a spontaneous emotional reaction, the action itself carried not only emotional but also social and cultural meaning; respectable women tore their faces as appropriate mourning at an honorable death. The Virgin Mary was the medieval mourner par excellence, and images of her grief at the foot of the cross emphasised mourning as women's work. In one of the *cantigas*, for example, a woman connects her own mourning to Mary's experience as a grieving mother, saying: 'Oh glorious Virgin, you who bore a Son for the salvation of the world and cared for him and nourished him and then, dear Lady, saw him killed and die a painful death, know how one who rears a child grieves'.[13] Castilian writer Gonzalo de Berceo (d. 1264) depicts the Virgin Mary herself tearing her hair and rending her cheeks in his *El duelo de la Virgen*, and Mary and the other women mourners appear in similar states of extreme bodily mourning throughout *planctus Mariae* poetry.[14]

Despite its omnipresence in narrative and artistic sources, cheek rending actually held a somewhat ambivalent status, both prescribed and proscribed.[15] On a local level, many municipal legal codes, or *fueros*, explicitly restricted forms of perceived excessive mourning. For example, the 13th-century Fuero de Zamora prohibits any man or woman from tearing themselves or their clothing, from singing laments and from wearing mourning clothes, except a son for his father, a vassal for his lord, a wife for her husband, or a husband for his wife.[16] Similarly, the 13th-century Fuero de Soria restricts the self-mutilation of excessive mourning, prohibiting any man from tearing himself and allowing women to tear themselves only at the death of their husbands.[17] These regulations allow some types of

---

[13] *Cantiga* 241, Kulp-Hill (2000: 291–292).

[14] For an analysis of Mary's bodily gestures of mourning in *El duelo de la Virgen*, see Del Campo (2015: 311–326). On women and gestures of mourning in other *planctus Mariae* works, see Muñoz Fernández (2006).

[15] The same is true in early medieval Islamic culture; on cheek rending and restrictions on women's mourning, see Halevi (2004: 3–39; 2007: 114–142).

[16] Fuero de Zamora 87: 'Esta es postura que el conseyo de Çamora puso que nengun omne nin ne[n]guna mugier non se messe nin se carpa nin faga xanto, nin ponga lucho, salvo fiyo por padre, o vassalo por senor, o mugier por marido, o marido por muggier'. Majada Neila (1983: 49). An early version of this *fuero* was granted in 1062, a semi-extensive version was confirmed by Alfonso IX in 1208, and the above edition comes from a 1289 redaction.

[17] Fuero de Soria 315: 'Por foyr del mal (et) dela tristeza ninguno varones njn mugieres non sean osados de messar sobre defunto njnguno. Otrosi las mugieres que se non messen, salvo

extreme mourning, but they implicitly restrict exactly the kind of mourning that is most prominent in the *Cantigas de Santa María,* that of mothers mourning for their children. While the law codes give no stated purpose for restricting cheek rending to certain circumstances, women weeping, wailing and tearing at their bloody cheeks would probably have been visible and perhaps disruptive to their entire communities. Children likely died more frequently than husbands; allowing women to tear their cheeks only at the deaths of their husbands might have reduced the overall public spectacle that even a single mourning woman would have made in a town.

Castilian royal law codes, including the *Siete Partidas*, compiled around 1265, also penalised acts of bodily mourning, ostensibly on the religious grounds that excessive mourning reflected a lack of faith in the hope of the resurrection and accomplished nothing for the dead.[18] Notably, Alfonso X of Castile both composed the *Cantigas de Santa María,* which presented cheek rending as a standard part of traditional mourning practices, and supervised and promulgated the *Siete Partidas,* which condemned and penalised cheek rending and other types of excessive mourning. This seeming contradiction, however, was standard throughout both Iberia and Italy; while ecclesiastical and legal authorities tried to limit excessive mourning, the actual practice of loud laments and the tearing of the hair, clothes and face continued relatively unabated throughout the medieval period.[19]

Scholars generally attribute these efforts to restrict the bodily performances of mourning to civic anxiety over the perceived instability of extreme emotion, and this could correlate with the association between mourning and madness in

---

la mugier por su maridom si quisiere; mas cada uno de sus oios llore quanto quisiere. Et las mugieres que non trayan llanto por la villa'. Sánchez (1919: 112). A *breve* version of this *fuero* was granted between 1109 and 1111 and an extensive version sometime after 1196; the above edition comes from a redacted version confirmed by Alfonso X in 1256.

[18] For this religious argument, see *Las Siete Partidas,* Partida I, Tit. IV, law XLIII, 'How Mourning for the Dead Is Not Beneficial, but Injurious', in Burns (2001: 35). This is a common theme among late antique and early medieval ecclesiastical writers; see Lansing (2008: 99–122). For other legal restrictions on excessive mourning in Iberia from the 13th through the 15th centuries, see Muñoz Fernández (2009: 111–118). For similar restrictions in Italian cities, see Hughes (1994).

[19] Ritual mourning practices persisted through the early modern period and, in some cases, even into the 20th century. Safran (2014: 133–134) notes that in southern Italy, 'such acts as tearing the hair and lacerating one's face continued to be proscribed at the local level' into the 17th century. Amelang (2005: 3–4) discusses Carlo Levi's reports of cheek rending and other actions of excessive mourning in northern Italy in 1935, and he problematizes the perceived continuity of traditional mourning practices in a static Mediterranean.

the *Cantigas de Santa María*.[20] In *cantiga* 168, a woman 'grieved so deeply for the last [child] who died that she almost went mad', and *cantiga* 21 describes a mother who not only tore her cheeks in grief at the loss of her son, she 'almost lost her mind'.[21] Another mother's grief for her son was 'so great that she went mad because of it, as many women do'.[22] One *cantiga* even portrays extreme grief as a kind of illness requiring miraculous healing; a mother whose child had died 'was so grief stricken that she lost her mind', and the miracle of the *cantiga* was not the resurrection of the child, who remained dead, but rather the healing of the mother from her mourning-induced madness.[23] The *cantigas* present the connection between mourning and madness as specifically gendered; while women commonly went mad from grief, men wept and grieved deeply but did not descend into madness.[24]

Restrictions on the physical gestures of mourning may be connected to larger ideas of civic stability, but they also seem to stem from a more specific fear of women's embodied mourning and their unrestrained emotion and sexuality.[25] Widows who had covered their hair since their weddings let it down in public, and they bared and even struck their breasts, turning symbols of marriage and motherhood into testaments of death. Women whose bodies had so carefully reflected their husbands' or fathers' honor and status through clothing, jewelry, and carefully applied cosmetics and perfumes now paraded in public humiliation and abjection, clawing at their hair and tearing their faces.[26] As Hughes argues, the 'undifferentiated body of mourning women' posed a particular challenge for cities that were trying to establish or maintain social order; these rituals reflected the inversion and upheaval of death, but they also could have been seen as potential incitements to other forms of social or political inversion and instability.[27] From a more religious standpoint, these kinds of gestures could be seen as heretical or faithless—disregarding the hope of the world to come—or as ostentatious displays

---

[20] For the connection between civic order and mourning restrictions, see Lansing (2008), especially 187–202. Lansing argues that laws restricting excessive grief in the Italian communes were part of a larger program to regulate male emotionality and promote civil order, and the *fueros*' restrictions on excessive grief might stem from a similar concern with the appearance of public order, especially in unstable or transitional frontier areas.

[21] Cantiga 168, Kulp-Hill (2000: 203); Cantiga 21, Kulp-Hill (2000: 30).

[22] Cantiga 168, Kulp-Hill (2000: 203); Cantiga 347, Kulp-Hill (2000: 422).

[23] Cantiga 331, Kulp-Hill (2000: 402).

[24] Instead, the *cantigas* tend to associate male madness with the devil.

[25] Hughes (1994: 32).

[26] On medieval Iberian women's health and cosmetics, see work by Cabré i Pairet (2000); also Caballero Navas (2008).

[27] Hughes (1994: 32).

of the flesh, meant to seduce unsuspecting men.²⁸ Late 4th-century church father John Chrysostom, for example, explicitly linked cheek rending and mourning to women's unrestrained sexuality. He condemned women who 'make a show of their mourning and lamentation: baring their arms, tearing their hair, making scratches down their cheeks', and he suggested that women often let loose their hair and tore their faces and clothing to 'attract the gaze of men' and 'attract lovers'.²⁹ The disruption of death unmoored women and their bodies from the constraints of Christian society, allowing them then to veer into madness, as in the *cantigas*, or into unbridled sexuality.

Cheek Rending as a Legal Act

In mourning, cheek rending appears alongside a range of interchangeable gestures used to refer to the entire ritual process of lament; in rape cases, it stands alone, and it takes on legal significance. Iberian sources use a variety of verbs to describe cheek rending as an act of mourning, including *rascar, grafinar, mesar, carpir, desfacer, cortar* and *romper*. All of these verbs have similar meanings—to scratch, to rip, to tear, to strip—and they are used in municipal legal codes, or *fueros,* as a requirement for women seeking to prosecute a claim of rape. Granted from the late 11th century and throughout the 12th and early 13th centuries, the *fueros extensos* derive from earlier *fueros breves* or *cartas pueblas*, which originally conceded royal or noble privileges to recently founded or conquered towns throughout Iberia. The *fueros* provided laws and legal procedures for each town before the advent of centralised royal law in the mid-13th century, and they were designed to attract new settlers and establish peace and stability as the Iberian Christian kingdoms fought their Muslim neighbors and expanded southward. These *fueros* are practical legal codes, without the overt ideological goals often found in royal law codes. The *fueros* can include hundreds of regulations on everyday matters, from which days Jews and Christians could use the bathhouses to how bakers should be fined for heating their public bread ovens badly, and the stipulations on rape and cheek rending should be read within this practical framework. Although not all of the *fueros* require cheek rending as proof of rape, the cheek-rending requirement appears so commonly in so many of the *fueros*, and especially in seemingly unrelated *fueros*, that it can be taken to represent the standard judicial procedure in 12th- and early 13th-century Iberia, particularly in Castile and León and in the Castilian Extremadura.³⁰

---

²⁸ Barasch (1976: 35–38).
²⁹ *In Ioannem Homiliae,* no. 62. Goggins (1959: 165–179, 174, 177).
³⁰ In her legal history of rape in Iberia, Rodríguez Ortiz (1997: 296) calls the requirement that women claw their cheeks as proof of rape 'sin duda alguna, el requisito más generalizado

The widely influential *fuero* of Cuenca, which was first granted by King Alfonso VIII of Castile between 1189 and 1193, survives today in three main redactions, two Latin and one Romance, and all three require cheek rending as proof of rape.[31] The *fuero* stipulates that a woman who had been raped should make her complaint to the *iudex* and the *alcalde* within three days, 'having clawed her cheeks'.[32] The language used here, generally *genas secatas,* cut cheeks, in Latin or *mexillas rascadas,* scratched cheeks, in Romance, changes only slightly throughout the Cuenca family of *fueros;* the *fueros* of Baeza, Béjar, Alcaraz, Alarcón, Alcázar, Iznatoraf, Plasencia and Zorita de los Canes sometimes substitute *sus fazes* or *la cara* for *mexillas,* cheeks, but the meaning remains the same throughout—the woman must publicly tear, claw or otherwise rend her cheeks as a prerequisite for bringing a valid accusation of rape. The *fueros* make clear that this cheek rending was separate from the assault itself—it was self-inflicted by the woman upon making her claim, and was not an injury incurred during the attack. Moreover, unlike the hue and cry required of rape victims in other areas of medieval Europe, cheek rending did not necessarily follow immediately after the assault and was not intended to help villagers apprehend a fleeing attacker; theoretically, a woman who had been raped had three days to decide whether or not to press charges and rend her cheeks. While cheek rending itself did not prove the fact of rape, it initiated the prosecutorial process and forced the accused man to respond to the claim.

Closely related to the Fuero de Cuenca, the Fuero de Teruel especially emphasises the absolute necessity of cheek rending for a woman seeking to make valid claim of rape, as both the Latin and Romance versions provide contrasting narratives of how this judicial process could proceed. If the woman did not come before the judge within three days *cum seccatis genis,* with clawed cheeks, her attacker did not have to respond to her claim; conversely, if she did appear before the judge within three days with clawed cheeks, the claim proceeded and the attacker was required to compensate her and her family according to the rubrics

---

en los fueros y, al mismo tiempo, más llamativo'. On rape in the *fueros,* see Dillard (1984: 181–192).

[31] The Forma Primordial survives in a mid-13th-century manuscript, the Forma Sistemática, in a manuscript dated to the 13th or 14th century. The Romance versions survive in a complete edition in the Codice Valentino, from the late 13th to early 15th centuries. The definitive modern edition of all three redactions is Ureña y Smenjaud (2003), which was the primary basis for James Powers's (2000) English translation.

[32] Powers (2000: 82). Forma Primordial, r. 277: 'habuerit genas secatas'. Forma Sistemática, r. 206: 'habens genas seccatas'. Códice Valentino, r. 21: 'tenjendo las mexillas rrascadas'. Ureña y Smenjaud (2003: 318–320).

on punishment for rape already outlined in the *fuero*.[33] Likewise, at Alba de Tormes, a raped woman was required to come to the nearest town *carpiendo y rascando*, tearing and scratching; if she did not come in this way, *si assi non uinere,* her claim could not proceed.[34] In Viguera and Val de Funes, in Navarre, the same principle applied; if a raped woman did not rend her cheeks, *si non rascare sus faces,* she was judged together with her attacker for adultery or fornication.[35]

The primary concern of all the *fueros* that deal with questions of rape was the will of the woman involved and the credibility of her claim.[36] For example, the titles for the laws on rape in the Fuero de Cuenca focus not on the crime itself but on whether or not the woman should be believed. Although the Romance version of the Fuero de Cuenca has 'Dela muger forçada o rrascada', both Latin versions use the title 'Que mulier de opressione credatur', or what woman should be believed concerning violation.[37] Likewise, the *fueros* of Iznatoraf, Alcaraz, Baeza and Zorita de los Canes use almost equivalent language—'Qual mugier deue seer creyda por forçada', which woman should be believed concerning rape.[38] If the woman was forced against her will, if the attack occurred 'non per sue voluntud', then the attacker could be prosecuted and the woman found innocent, but if she consented in any way she was disinherited and exiled as an enemy, together with the accused man.[39]

The underlying assumption, as Heath Dillard demonstrates, is that women did run away with men voluntarily, that illicit sex was more likely to be adultery or fornication than rape, and that abduction might really be a cover for clandestine marriage.[40] Elopement was a persistent problem in frontier towns, especially

---

[33] Fuero de Teruel, r. 364: Caruana Gómez de Barreda (1974: 317–318) and Castañé Llinás (1989: 518–519). Fuero de Teruel, Romance, r. 476: Gorosch (1950: 295).
[34] Fuero de Alba de Tormes, r. 21: Castro and Onís (1916: 301–302).
[35] Fuero de Viguera y Val de Funes, r. 39: Ramos y Loscertales (1956: 11).
[36] Robertson (2001: 285) argues that the focus on consent and the violation of the will in rape assumes and even emphasises the individual subjectivity of the raped woman.
[37] Ureña y Smenjaud (2003: 318–320); Powers (2000: 82).
[38] Fuero de Baeza, r. 249. Roudil (1962: 106).
[39] Fueros de Usagre and Cáceres, r. 73: Ureña y Smenjaud and Bonilla y San Martin (1907: 27). Phillips (2000: 125) argues that while modern law on rape is based on the idea of the 'unconsenting will', medieval conceptions of rape focus more on the 'assaulted body'; while this might be true in English legal sources, I do not see this to have been the case in Iberia, at least in the 12th and 13th centuries. Later legislation on rape emphasises marks of physical resistance on the assaulted body, but the bodily emphasis in the *fueros* points not to resistance but to the woman's desire to prove nonconsent, as the injuries are self-inflicted rather than incurred during the assault itself.
[40] Dillard (1984: 134–147).

because women were scarce and an ecclesiastically valid marriage could be contracted through consent alone without parental approval; abduction, whether initially forceful or voluntary, often led to valid marriage.[41] The task of the raped woman, then, was to prove that she had not eloped and regretted her decision, but that she had been attacked 'aforcia e sin su grado', by force and without her consent.[42] The task of the *fueros* was to provide justice for genuine victims of rape while discouraging false accusations in circumstances in which women consented to illicit sex. The stakes were high, as the *fueros* set out harsh penalties for both rape and false accusations, and the judges and *alcaldes* who enforced the *fueros* faced the nearly impossible task of determining the inner mental state of the accusing woman.[43] The social or emotional function of cheek rending may explain why individual women tore their cheeks after being raped, but not why the *fueros* required and accepted cheek rending as legal proof.[44] Why, then, would the *fueros* require women who had been raped to rend their cheeks? How did the physical action of tearing the face function not merely as a sign of grief or distress, but as a valid form of legal proof?

One provision in the *fuero* of Viguera and Val de Funes offers a possible explanation, and a connection between cheek rending as mourning and cheek rending as proof. If an *infancona* (noble woman) accused of marrying a *villano* (non-noble townsman) tore her face in grief after his death, this action affirmed the marriage as valid and the woman took his lower status, becoming a non-noble *villana* for the rest of her life.[45] Here, the act of cheek rending in grief demonstrates the inner reality of the marriage; even if the woman verbally denied the marriage, the physical sign of her torn cheeks spoke for her, and the cheek rending enacted what was already essentially true. This perceived ability of cheek rending to make

---

[41] Dillard (1984: 141).

[42] Fuero de Ledesma, r. 191: Castro and de Onís (1916: 249–250).

[43] In her discussion of rape cases in Perpignan in the late 13th century, Rebecca Lynn Winer also emphasises the near impossibility of proving a rape claim; Winer argues that the unreasonably high burden of proof, as well as the social stigma that came even with proven rape, discouraged women from reporting rape and encouraged private settlements between the families of the victim and the attacker. Winer (2000: 173–174, 177–189).

[44] The few scholars that mention cheek rending as proof of rape suggest that the gesture functioned as proof because it demonstrated the woman's internal mental anguish. See Dillard (1984: 184) and Córdoba de la Llave (1994: 55).

[45] Fuero de Viguera y Val de Funes, r. 272: 'Et si jnfancona fuere accusada que casó con villano e lo negare, e después se probare que fué por tres dias so hun techo con aquel omne, si no fuere en logar de toda gent, et el villano murjere et vinjere et [vinjere] ronpiere sus fazes, o su abrigadura pusiere en la cabeca, o si después de su muerte saylliere sobre la fuessa por IX dias continuos, será villana por siempre'. Ramos y Loscertales (1956: 51).

visible the otherwise inaccessible internal truth allows it to function effectively as proof in rape cases, in which the internal mental state of the woman lies at the very heart of the charge.

Moreover, this use of cheek rending in a legal sense underscores the potential legal significance of the gesture; cheek rending was a legal act, with significant legal repercussions. We might be able to understand cheek rending in this instance as functioning like a performative speech act; when performed under the right circumstances, cheek rending described but also fundamentally altered the social reality.[46] In rending her cheeks at her non-noble husband's burial, a noble *infancona* not only performed appropriate female grief, she actually transformed her legal status to match that of her dead husband. When a woman appeared in the plaza mayor of Cuenca tearing and scratching at her face, she performed the customary gestures of grief and distress, but she also initiated a legal process and, in a legal sense, *became* a victim of rape.

Cheek Rending as a Physical Gesture

Studies of medieval emotion and gesture have demonstrated that weeping was seen as a sign of sincerity, a physical and external expression of internal emotional pain or genuine repentance.[47] This connection between weeping and sincerity correlates with the emphasis in the *fueros* on the credibility of raped women, whose internal innocence was made manifest through external signs. Weeping would not have affected the body itself in nearly the same way as cheek rending, and the bodily aspect of cheek rending, both as part of mourning and as a legal act, cannot be overstated. The verbs used to describe the action of cheek rending –*rascar, grafinar, mesar, carpir, desfacer, cortar, romper*—signify real physical violence; the mourners scratch, rip, tear, cut and strip their faces. This is not a symbolic gesture. The *Primera Crónica General* offers a violent description of women mourners who tore and scratched their faces, 'tornandolas en sangre et en carne biva', stripping them back to blood and to open wounds.[48] Isidore of Seville (d. 636), whose work was read and recopied throughout the 12th and 13th centuries, associated cheek rending not with despair or even mourning, but with the crimson color of blood; in his explanation of the etymology of *sanguis* (blood), he argued that blood is the possession of a soul, and that therefore 'women will lacerate their cheeks in grief, and crimson robes and crimson flowers are offered to the

---

[46] On performative speech acts, see Austin (1962: 5–6).
[47] See Blanchfield (2012); also Blanchfield (1999).
[48] *Primera Crónica General*, cap. 1134, p. 773.

dead'.⁴⁹ Images of cheek rending as part of mourning are commonplace in funerary sculpture and art, and the gestures depicted are often violent and visceral.⁵⁰ Most arresting are the *Plañideros* paintings in the chapel of San Andrés de Mahamud in Burgos.⁵¹ These four small wooden panels, which were commissioned in 1295 and would originally have been affixed to the front of the coffins of Sancho Sánchez Carillo and his wife, Juana, depict male and female mourners tearing at their cheeks, foreheads and hair. The mourners' mouths are closed, and they appear to express their grief primarily through their bodies and their physical actions.⁵² Most importantly for understanding cheek rending as a physical gesture, these brightly colored images clearly show red lines on the mourners' cheeks and foreheads.

Written sources underscore the physical and visible effects of cheek rending on the body. The *Siete Partidas* even associates cheek rending with disfigurement; a law on punishment for those who mourn for the dead defines mourning as 'romper las caras por los muertos e desfigurarlas', to tear the face for the dead and to disfigure it.⁵³ Moreover, this same law specifically mentions the physical marks that cheek rending would leave on the face, and it even forbids priests from administering the sacraments until mourners 'fuessen sanos de las señales que ouiessen fecho en sus caras', until they were healed from the marks which they had made on their faces.⁵⁴ This suggests that cheek rending left real, visible marks, that their bodies were literally marked, and possibly even scarred, with grief. The *Libro de los Fueros de Castilla*, a collection of Castilian royal law compiled between 1248 and 1252, may refer to similar marks, as it specifically excludes the marks made by cheek rending in its list of injuries for which women could receive

---

[49] Isidore of Seville, *Etymologies*, XI.I.123; translated in Barney et al. (2006: 239).
[50] Cheek rending is also frequently depicted in art and sculpture representing the biblical Massacre of the Innocents, in which mothers tear their cheeks in mourning over the deaths of their infant children. On mourning gestures in medieval Iberian art, see Miguélez Cavero (2007); also Miguélez Cavero (2015: 35–62).
[51] The *Plañideros* panels are currently in Sala 19 of the Museu Nacional d'Art de Cataluyna, in Barcelona, inventory numbers 004372-003, 004372-004, 004372-005 and 004372-006. See Gutiérrez Baños (2005: t. II, 101–109 [núm. 32], 386–401), cited in San José Alonso (2010: 203).
[52] Other tombs with similar images of mourning include those of Blanca of Navarre (1156) in Nájera, Esteban Domingo (1261) in Ávila, and the Infante Felipe and his wife in Villalcázar de Sirga. See Del Campo (2015: 310–311). The sepulcher of Bishop Gonzalo de Hinojosa (d. 1237) in the Capilla de San Gregorio, Catedral de Burgos, contains similar images of monks tearing their faces.
[53] Partida 1, Tit. IV, law XLIV: Burns (2001: 172).
[54] Partida 1, Tit. IV, law XLIV. Another manuscript has the same law specifically banning the sacraments from 'los que rompiesen sus faces rascándose', those who tear their faces, scratching them. See Burns (2001: 172).

compensation. Women could be compensated for wounds caused by knives, rocks, wooden instruments or any other prohibited item, but not for injuries which the *alcalde* could see were scratched with the fingernails ('rascunno de hunna').[55] While this law could refer to scratches incurred during some kind of fight or assault, there is no similar regulation of scratch marks for men; scratching and tearing with the fingernails seems to be specifically associated with women and with women's bodies, and the marks left by tearing the skin are assumed to be visible to a presiding *alcalde*.

Medical texts also reference the physical marks left by cheek rending. The 12th-century medical treatise *De curis mulierum* (Treatments for Women), which was included in the Salernian *Trotula* text, describes an ointment which the women of Salerno used 'contra maculas in facie quas faciunt salernitane pro mortuis', to treat the marks on their faces which they made in mourning for the dead.[56] Another version of the same text refers to the ointment as 'contra crustulas pro mortuis factas', for the scabs made by mourning for the dead.[57] If women commonly tore their cheeks in ritual mourning for the dead, as the Iberian sources overwhelmingly illustrate, they would then have to deal with the wounds, scabs and scars left by this self-mutilation. Moreover, these wounds would have marked the most visible part of the women's bodies—their faces. Iberian medical and cosmetic texts suggest that women from all levels of society likely had some access to knowledge or even recipes concerning skin conditions, blemishes and treatments, and women probably would have shared knowledge of how to heal the marks left from cheek rending. Moreover, as regulations on mourning in the *Siete Partidas* suggest, women might have had religious motivations in seeking to heal their scars, as they could be excluded from the sacraments—effectively excommunicated—until these marks had healed.

While further research into medieval Iberian medical texts, many of which include discussions of beauty and recipes for women's cosmetics and skin treatments, may uncover more strategies for how women dealt with the physical marks left behind by cheek rending, it is clear that cheek rending cannot be divorced from its effect on real bodies and real faces. If the physical actions of cheek rending as mourning and as legal act were the same, as the use of similar

---

[55] Sánchez (1924: r. 5, p. 30).
[56] *De curis mulierum,* section 167: Green (2001: 224, n. 164). This is from the version of the *De curis mulierum* text that circulated independently and is closest in form to what it must have looked like when it was first written in Salerno.
[57] *De curis mulierum,* section 167, proto-ensemble text: Green (2001: 241, n. 32). The standardised ensemble text has 'contra coraculas uel catharactas pro mortuis factas', for the cataracts and rivulets made in mourning for the dead. See Green (2001: 241, n. 32).

vocabulary suggests, then a widow and a raped woman would both bear similar marks on their faces. It makes some sense that women who had been raped would perform the same ritual actions of grief and distress as did women mourning for the dead; in fact, cheek rending as proof of rape has been overwhelmingly interpreted as an expression of grief and distress. Cheek rending was not an involuntary or natural gesture, however, but rather a conscious decision; in mourning, women chose to rend their cheeks and therefore perform the appropriate gestures of female grief. One might imagine a woman who chose not to rend her cheeks at the death of her husband in order to preserve her noble status, or a mother who chose not to rend her cheeks at the death of a child to avoid being penalised by her local town council. In cases of rape, women tore their cheeks as a legal act. A woman could rend her cheeks as part of a false rape accusation, as described above in *cantiga* 355, without any internal grief or distress; conversely, a woman who had been raped could decide to hide the assault and not press charges by declining to rend her cheeks. Women tore their cheeks not only out of emotional pain, but because the gesture itself conveyed social meaning and bore legal significance.

The physical act of cheek rending, and the facial marks that it left behind, connect mourning and rape in more than just the expression of grief and distress. Rape could be understood as a kind of death, but also as a disruption to the expected life progression of marriage, sex and children. Scholarship on Roman funeral ritual has emphasised women's role in mourning as maintaining a connection between birth and death; women regulated passage both into and out of the world of the living, and the sexual body that mourned dead fathers, husbands and children also brought new life into the world.[58] In medieval Iberia, this same mourning body was seen as explicitly sexual, and a woman tearing her clothing and rending her cheeks might closely resemble a woman claiming to have been raped. Furthermore, facial mutilation has long been linked to sex; in the early medieval period women could suffer facial mutilation as a punishment for sexual offenses, and women are reported to have voluntarily mutilated their faces as a deterrent to sexual assault.[59] For women who had already been assaulted, disfiguring the face might have been a means of claiming their innocence after the fact. Whether or not the actual cheek rending left permanent scars, it would certainly have marked the woman within her community; Skinner argues that even hair cutting, while not permanently disfiguring, could have as profound a symbolism within the community as a more

---

[58] See, for example, Corbeill (2004: 67–106).
[59] On gender and facial mutilation generally, see Skinner (2017: 133–158). See also Skinner (2015: 187–189) and Tibbetts Schulenburg (1986); on Abbess Ebba and Anglo-Saxon nuns mutilating themselves to avoid being raped by Vikings, see Horner (2001: 120).

permanent disfiguration, like cutting the nose or gouging the eyes.[60] In the small towns in 12th- and 13th-century Castile and León, the entire community would have seen, or at least heard about, a woman publicly rending her cheeks, and the woman's experiences, either as a widow or as a victim of rape, would remain apparent on her face until the wounds healed or the scars faded. Furthermore, both rape and widowhood marked a profound change in a woman's status, even though both processes occurred completely outside of the woman's control. When a grieving wife tore her cheeks, she gave physical expression to her new status as a widow rather than a wife, but she also performed the traditional and honorable role of a mourning wife, as there was honor and dignity in the appropriate and expected humiliation of mourning. When a raped woman tore her cheeks, she gave visible and physical expression to the often invisible violence of rape, and she visibly demonstrated the shame and disgrace of her violation.[61] At the same time, this cheek rending also vindicated her, restoring her to the honor of innocence, as she became not an adulteress but a victim of force. Rather than testifying verbally, a raped woman demonstrated the reality of her violation through the self-mutilation of her physical body, which then testified for her. Iberian municipal law constructed legal truth through oaths, witness swearing, ordeals and documentary evidence; in cases of rape, the law constructed truth through women's bodily performances. The gesture of cheek rending, then, spoke not just the emotional truth of mourning, but also legal truth.

Bibliography

Amelang, J. 2005. Mourning becomes eclectic: Ritual lament and the problem of continuity. *Past and Present* 187: 3–31.

Austin, J. L. 1962. *How to Do Things with Words.* Cambridge (MA): Harvard University Press.

Barasch, M. 1976. *Gestures of Despair in Medieval and Early Renaissance Art.* New York: New York University Press.

Barney, S. A., Lewis, W. J., Beach, J. A., and Berghof, O. 2006. *The Etymologies of Isidore of Seville.* Cambridge: Cambridge University Press.

Barton, S. and Fletcher, R. (eds) 2000. *The World of El Cid: Chronicles of the Spanish Reconquest.* Manchester: Manchester University Press, St. Martin's Press.

Blanchfield, L. A. 1999. The sincere body: The performance of weeping and emotion in Late Medieval Italian sermons. *Quidditas* 20: 117–135.

---

[60] Skinner (2017: 139).

[61] For example, the Fuero de Jaca requires a woman not only to rend her cheeks, but to 'dire e mostrar sa onta', declare and show her shame or disgrace. Molho (1964: 61).

Blanchfield, L. A. 2012. Prolegomenon: Considerations of weeping and sincerity in the Middle Ages, in E. Gertsman (ed.), *Crying in the Middle Ages: Tears of History*: xxi–xxx. New York: Routledge.

Burns, R. I. S. J. (ed.) 2001. *Las Siete Partidas,* vol. 1: *The Medieval Church: The World of Clerics and Laymen.* Philadelphia: University of Pennsylvania Press.

Caballero Navas, C. 2008. The care of women's health and beauty: An experience shared by Medieval Jewish and Christian women. *Journal of Medieval History* 34(2): 146–163.

Cabré i Pairet, M. 2000. From a master to a laywoman: A feminine manual of self-help. *Dynamis: Acta Hispanica ad Medicinae Scientiarumque Historiam Illustrandam* 20: 371–393.

Caruana Gómez de Barreda, J. 1974. *El Fuero Latino de Teruel.* Teruel: Instituto de Estudios Turolenses.

Castañé Llinás, J. 1989. *El Fuero de Teruel: Edición crítica con introducción y traducción.* Teruel: Ayuntamiento de Teruel.

Castro, A. and de Onís, F. 1916. *Fueros Leoneses de Zamora, Salamanca, Ledesma, y Alba de Tormes.* Madrid: Imprenta de los Sucesores de Hernando.

Corbeill, A. 2004. *Nature Embodied, Gesture in Ancient Rome.* Princeton (NJ): Princeton University Press.

Córdoba de la Llave, R. 1994. *El instinto diabólico: agresiones sexuales en la Castilla medieval.* Córdoba: Universidad de Córdoba.

Del Campo, A. 2015. Crying tears, tearing clothes: Expressing grief and rage in the Middle Ages, in F. Sabaté (ed.) *Life and Religion in the Middle Ages*: 305-326. Newcastle upon Tyne: Cambridge Scholars Publishing.

Desamparados Cabanes Pecourt, M. 1964. *La Crónica latina de los reyes de Castilla: edición crítica e indices,* Textos Medievales 11. Valencia: J. Nácher.

Dillard, H. 1984. *Daughters of the Reconquest: Women in Castilian Town Society, 1100-1300.* Cambridge: Cambridge University Press.

Goggins, T. A. (trans.) 1959. *Commentary on Saint John the Apostle and Evangelist, Homilies 48-88.* Washington (DC): Catholic University of America Press.

Gorosch, M. 1950. *El Fuero de Teruel.* Stockholm: Uppsala.

Green, M. (ed.) 2001. *The Trotula: A medieval compendium of women's medicine.* Philadelphia: University of Pennsylvania Press.

Gutiérrez Baños, F. 2005. *Aportación al estudio de la pintura de estilo gótico lineal en Castilla y León: precisiones cronológicas y corpus de pintura mural y sobre table.* Madrid: Fundación Universitaria Española.

Halevi, L. 2004. Wailing for the dead: The role of women in early Islamic funerals. *Past and Present* 183: 3–39.

Halevi, L. 2007. *Muhammad's Grave: Death Rites and the Making of Islamic Society.* New York: Columbia University Press.

Horner, S. 2001. *The Discourse of Enclosure: Representing Women in Old English Literature.* New York: State University of New York.
Kulp-Hill, K. (trans.) 2000. *Songs of Holy Mary of Alfonso X, the Wise: A Translation of the Cantigas de Santa María.* Tempe: Arizona Center for Medieval and Renaissance Studies.
Lansing, C. 2008. *Passion and Order: Restraint of Grief in the Medieval Italian Communes.* Ithaca: Cornell University Press.
Majada Neila, J. 1983. *Fuero de Zamora: introducción, transcripción, vocabulario.* Salamanca: Librería Cervantes.
Menéndez Pidal, R. (ed.) 1906. *Primera Crónica General. Estoria de España que mandó componer Alfonso el Sabio y se continuaba bajo Sancho IV en 1289. Tomo I: Texto.* Madrid: Bailly-Baillière e Hijos.
Mettmann, W. (ed.) 1964. *Cantigas de Santa María,* vol. 3. Coimbra: Universidade de Coimbra.
Miguélez Cavero, A. 2007. *Actitudes gestuales en la iconografía del románico peninsular hispano: el sueño, el dolor espiritual y otras expresiones similares.* León: Universidad de León.
Miguélez Cavero, A. 2015. Gesto, imagen y liturgia: las representaciones de dolor y lamento en la escultura funeraria portuguesa (siglos XII–XIV), in C. Varela Fernandes, *Imagens e liturgia na Idade Média:* 35–62. Moscavide: Secretariado Nacional para os Bens Culturais da Igreja.
Molho, M. (ed.) 1964. *El Fuero de Jaca: Edición crítica.* Zaragoza: Instituto de Estudios Pirenaicos.
Muñoz Fernández, A. 2006. 'Planctus Mariae': Mujeres, lágrimas y agencia cultural. *Arenal. Revista de Historia de las Mujeres* 13(2): 237–261.
Muñoz Fernández, A. 2009. Llanto, palabras y gestos. La muerte y el duelo en el mundo medieval hispánico (morfología ritual, agencias culturales y controversias). *Cuadernos de historia de España* 83: 107–40.
Owen Hughes, D. 1994. Mourning rites, memory, and civilization in premodern Italy, in J. Chiffoleau, L. Martines, and A. Paravicini Bagliani (eds), *Riti e rituali nelle società medievali*: 23–38. Spoleto: Centro Italiano di Studi sull'Alto Medioevo.
Phillips, K. M. 2000. Written on the body: Reading rape from the twelfth to the fifteenth centuries, in N. J. Menuge (ed.), *Medieval Women and the Law*: 125–144. Woodbridge: Boydell Press.
Powers, J. (trans.) 2000. *The Code of Cuenca: Municipal Law on the Twelfth-Century Castilian Frontier.* Philadelphia: University of Pennsylvania Press.
Ramos y Loscertales, J. M. 1956. *Fuero de Viguera y Val de Funes (edición crítica).* Salamanca: University of Salamanca.
Robertson, E. 2001. Public bodies and psychic domains: Rape, consent, and female subjectivity in Geoffrey Chaucer's *Troilus and Criseyde*, in E. Robertson and C.M.

Rose (eds), *Representing Rape in Medieval and Early Modern Literature*: 281–310. New York: Palgrave.

Rodríguez Ortiz, V. 1997. *Historia de la violación: Su regulación jurídica hasta fines de la Edad Media*. Madrid: Comunidad de Madrid.

Roudil, J. 1962. *El Fuero de Baeza: Edición, estudio y vocabulario*. The Hague: van Goor Zonen.

Safran, L. 2014. *The Medieval Salento: Art and Identity in Southern Italy*. Philadelphia: University of Pennsylvania Press.

San José Alonso, J. 2010. Restauración real, restauración virtual. Los templos de Santa María de Valbuena, en San Bernardo y de San Andrés en Mahamud. *Biblioteca: Estudio e Investigación* 25: 187–204.

Sánchez Alonso, B. (ed.) 1924. *Crónica del Obispo Don Pelayo*. Madrid: Imprenta de los Sucesores de Hernando.

Sánchez, G. (ed.) 1924. *Libro de los Fueros de Castiella*. Barcelona: Universidad de Barcelona.

Sánchez, G. 1919. *Fueros Castellanos de Soria y Alcalá de Henares*. Madrid: Imprenta de los Sucesores de Hernando.

Scarborough, C. L. 2012. Women as victims and criminals in the *Siete Partidas*, in A. Classen and C. L. Scarborough (eds), *Crime and Punishment in the Middle Ages and Early Modern Age: Mental-Historical Investigations of Basic Human Problems and Social Response*: 225–246. Berlin: de Gruyter.

Skinner, P. 2015. Marking the face, curing the soul? Reading the disfigurement of women in the Later Middle Ages, in N.K. Yoshikawa (ed.), *Medicine, Religion and Gender in Medieval Culture*: 181–201. Woodbridge: Boydell and Brewer.

Skinner, P. 2017. *Living with Disfigurement in the Middle Ages*. New York: Palgrave Macmillan.

Tibbetts Schulenburg, J. 1986. The heroics of virginity: Brides of Christ and sacrificial mutilation, in M.B. Rose (ed.) *Women in the Middle Ages and Renaissance: Literary and Historical Perspectives*: 29–72. Syracuse (NY): Syracuse University Press.

Ureña y Smenjaud, R. de 2003. *El Fuero de Cuenca (formas primitiva y sistemática: texto Latino, texto Castellano y adaptación del Fuero de Isnatoraf)*. Cuenca: Ediciones de la Universidad de Castilla-La Mancha.

Ureña y Smenjaud, R. and Bonilla y San Martin, A. 1907. *Fuero de Usagre, siglo XIII; anotado con las variants del de Cáceres*. Madrid: Hijos de Reus.

Winer, R. L. 2000. Defining rape in medieval Perpignan: Women plaintiffs before the law. *Viator* 31: 173–174, 177–189.

Clerical Leprosy and the Ecclesiastical Office: Dis/Ability and Canon Law

Ninon Dubourg

Leprosy (*lepra*)[1] is a chronic and infectious disease which has long-lasting disabling consequences for the sufferer. It affects mainly the peripheral nervous system and the skin, provoking a disastrous loss of sensation in various body parts and ultimately even the loss of limbs. The Old Testament (Leviticus 21:13–14) nominates priests as chiefly responsible for dealing with lepers, a descriptor which often referred to those suffering not just leprosy, but incurable skin diseases, or those deemed to be 'unclean'. What happens when a cleric contracts leprosy himself? How is clerical leprosy treated, and by whom? In such cases, as we shall see, the clerical hierarchy acts to contain the leprous cleric's apparent impurity.

Some contemporaries and historians deemed leprosy as a test in the name of God's love for redemption. On the contrary, some regarded it as proof of the Lord's damnation, to punish someone or the person's parents.[2] This ambiguity was stronger than for any other disease, because 'the cause and spread of the disease was little understood'.[3] In the 12th century, the Book of Job seemed to provide a favourable explanation for the disease,[4] since being sick was viewed as a consequence of being touched by the grace of God. Lazarus, the patron saint of many leper colonies, embodied this explanation because he epitomised 'the virtuous poor' for Christians. Nevertheless, this positive view shifted many times during the Middle Ages. For example, in the *Decretum Gratiani*, composed in two parts sometime around 1147[5], the father of canon law, Gratian, used *lepra* as a synonym for sin. This indiscriminate comingling of sin and leprosy was made clear in medieval times when leprosy was usually defined as a physical illness

---

[1] The Latin word *infirmitas* was often used to describe leprosy in medieval documents, revealing that it was the epitome of a disease with a universal significance. However, we can assume that in the papal letters I used as sources, *lepra* refers to the actual leprosy (called Hansen's disease), which seemed to be well diagnosed during the Middle Ages according to Demaitre (2007).
[2] Jeanne (2014: 69).
[3] Marcombe (2003: 140).
[4] Bériou and Touati (1991: 34).
[5] Winroth (2004).

resulting from loose morals.⁶ Because of the specificity of this disease, historians believed for a long time that lepers were excluded from medieval society, either quarantined in leper colonies or as beggars socially rejected with their ratchet.⁷ In most recent historiography, scholars tend to avoid using the notion of exclusion when analysing leprosy in the Middle Ages. Instead, critics analyse this relative ostracism as a different kind of social integration.⁸

I follow, and extend, this theoretical approach to medieval leprosy in this article and analyse the social consequences—both positive and negative—of a diagnosis of leprosy for a cleric. My study is focused on the specific issue of the ecclesiastical office for a leprous cleric, as a means to examine the wider issue of clerical leprosy. When a man entered the clergy, he held an ecclesiastical office and performed a number of spiritual duties attached to it (sometimes a cure of souls). The clerics, secular or regular, could also have a benefice attached to their ecclesiastical office in order to provide them a livelihood, but I will focus my analysis more on the social role they ensured, between the representation on the members of the secular (in case of *cura animarum*) or regular community (because of their leadership role), and their physical capacity to perform the tasks attached to their ecclesiastical office. My study shows that when a cleric was leprous, the papal chancery had many ways to manage his integration with regard to his subsequent (in)ability to hold an ecclesiastical office, specifically in the case of specific offices (as bishop or abbot) or for those with a *cura animarum*. I draw from the *Decretals of Gregory IX* and other canon laws, supplication letters and papal dispensation letters to see how leprous clerics were treated by the popes and the papal chancery in the 13th and 14th centuries. I will show that the exclusion was not the path chosen by the papal chancery for the leper-clerics and that it was preferable to offer them a relative social inclusion rather than an exclusion of the clergy. First, I examine the ecclesiastical interdiction against being both a leper and a cleric. Then, I consider the real problems leprosy would have caused for a

---

⁶ For the Latin text, see Richter and Friedberg (1879: 2), c. 1, Q. 1, c. 14, 'Cum ordinaretur episcopus, quod dedit aurum fuit, quod perdidit anima fuit; cum alium ordinaret, quod accepit aurum fuit, quod dedit lepra fuit' (Whom give the ordination to a bishop against money will lost his soul, whom give the order to someone else and accept money for it will be stroke by leprosy. The French translation (Löfstedt 1993: 9: 'qui ordene aucun par deniers, il ne li donne pas grace mes pechié') saves only the sinful idea and not the leprosy: 'whom give the order against money don't give him grave but sin'.
⁷ Ratchets are the noise-making devices lepers had to carry in order to make people aware of their presence. Historians previously thought that these devices were used to allow people to escape from the lepers, but the most recent historiography now promotes the ratchet as a tool to attract passers-by in order to receive alms from them.
⁸ Tabuteau (2012).

cleric's ability to fulfil his social role. Finally, I analyse the professional, spatial and social consequences of the disease when a leper was also a member of the clergy.

The Ecclesiastical Idea of Perfection

Canon law codified the core teachings of the Church, including rules for the clergy. However, canon law also established mechanisms by which the Church could issue letters of dispensation for some clerics, thereby allowing them to disobey the edicts of canon law without being found at fault. This study takes both canon law and dispensation letters into account as primary sources for examining how the Church went against its own rules about leper-clerics with dispensation letters. Such letters were issued by the Roman Catholic Church as a response to supplication letters written by the leprous cleric himself, his hierarchy or a lay or clerical informer. They formulated the cleric's requests for a special dispensation in order to contravene canon law—with regard to income or religious practices—necessitated by the circumstances of his disability (here, leprosy). Both supplication and dispensation letters offer us only partial insight into each case, literally as one side of a dialogue between at least two people or groups, the leper-cleric and his supporters or detractors and the Church. Often, it is impossible to know how the story ended, in part, at least, because of the quantity of letters sent and received and the poor organisational structures to deal with them. Nevertheless, the popes since the Gregorian Reform centralised the reception of all *causae majores* of the Church,[9] and so the papal chancery kept a great number of these letters in the chancery registers. In the centuries studied in this essay, and since the 12th century, the popes' decisions were absolute and, above all, by means of their high power of grace and the *plenitudo potestatis*.

Why was clerical leprosy such a problem? In a nutshell, clerics had to be perfect physically, like Christ. First, physical perfection was linked with moral perfection. These two impairments to enter the cleric condition put the applicant in situation of irregularity, for being outside the canonical norms. These canonical norms evolved over time. At the beginning of Christianity, moral perfection was a more important criterion than physical perfection because that last was just supposed to illustrate the moral wrongs.[10] But this matter of facts changed

---

[9] Gregory VII's *Dictatus Papae* is a commentary on the Gregorian Reform—Propositions XXI et VII.
[10] This idea was first expressed in several oft-quoted verses from Leviticus 21:16–24, translated into English in the Wycliffe Bible in the late 14th century: 'Nor shall he come to do his service; nor, as well, if he is blind, or lame; or too small, or too big; if he hath a crippled, or deformed, hand or foot; if he hath a botch, or a bulge, on his back; either if he

with the first canonical legislation (fourth and fifth centuries) because canonists distinguish *defectus infamiae*, which forbid ordination, and *defectus corporis*, which can prevent a man from entering the clergy.[11] To finish, in the canonical collections of the 12th and 13th centuries, physical perfection became a category of defects of the same gravity as moral ones. So, canon law, which fixed the rules and the means to go against itself, seized the question of the disabled clerics. The first important canonical collection to address this issue directly, the *Decretum Gratiani*, stated in several *distinctio* that a physically altered man could not be a member of the clergy.[12] Church councils could also legislate on infirmity. For example, less than a century after the composition of Gratian's legal textbook, canon 10 of the Fourth Council of the Lateran allowed a physically disabled bishop to send another cleric to do his normal clerical duties in his diocese.[13] Twenty years later, the *Decretals of Gregory IX* outlined in several chapters the rationale behind the disqualification of individuals from the clergy if they exhibited physical abnormalities.[14] Gregory claimed that the diseased simply could not enter major orders on a moral basis: the sinful nature of the disabled or diseased body prevented a cleric from performing routine duties, such as blessing the sacrament and leading the mass.[15]

The construction of the legal notion of *defectus corporis* by canon law implies that an infirmity could prevent the cleric from being ordinate or holding an ecclesiastical office. But, it is clear in the canonical texts mentioned above that an infirmity became a *defectus corporis* solely when the representation (*claritas*) of the minister and his physical capacities were questioned.[16] However, only a superior authority, like episcopal courts and more specifically the papal court, could judge if an infirmity led to these social consequences on representation and physical capacities. Thus, this perfection had to be checked before the priest's ordination, to prove his ability to hold an ecclesiastical office. This verification may not have been done systematically for all clerical appointments (especially to enter minor orders), but was frequently requested in suspected cases of leprosy. As in lay trials on leprosy, conducted when there was a suspicious case of leprosy within the

---

is bleary-eyed; if he hath white colour, or a pearl, in his eye, that hindereth his sight; if he hath a continual scab; if he hath a dry scab on his body; either if he be bruised in the privy members'. Noble, Wycliffe and Purvey (2010: 172). In Latin, see Weber, Gryson and Fischer (2007: 231).

[11] Guaydier (1933).
[12] Richter and Friedberg (1879), distinctio 55, c. 1–13; 34, c. 10; 36, c. 1; 49, c. 1.
[13] Mansi (1961: 998).
[14] Richter and Friedberg (1881), I–IX, Cap. 1, 9, 10, 15; I–XX, Cap. 1–7; III–VI, Cap. 1–5.
[15] To see all canonical legislation on leprosy, see Merzbacher (1967).
[16] Aquinas et al. (2005), Commentary on the Sentences by St Thomas Aquinas, IV, D. 25, Q. 2, art. 2.

society, an inquiry was launched after an individual was denounced. This element of denunciation is also connected to the role of *fama publica* (public reputation) and scandal (analysed in depth below), which launched the inquiry process.[17] For example, Theobaldus, treasurer of Rouen's superiors, specifically requested an examination after he was denounced as leprous:[18] "We order an examination of Theobaldi the treasurer of Rouen's election because some people insinuate that Theobaldi is infected by lepra. This is why we ask you [(Gervasio) bishop of Séez, the major archdeacon of Reims and the deacon of Amiens] to lead, under the invocation of the divine judgment firmly enjoining, an investigation made by the most faithful and honest medical experts."[19] Honorius III ordered this examination to silence people with a medical test administered by both lawyers and doctors, comparable to what would have happened in a lay trial. However, he asked for judges who were the most learned scholars in the field of medical investigation and who worked the most meticulously. In another letter, dated 18 May 1222, Honorius III, using his papal authority, allowed Theobaldus's ecclesiastic community to elect another 'appropriate' (*idoneus*)—i.e., definitely healthy—cleric, to celebrate mass whilst the investigation went on.[20]

Within the pontificate of John XXII, during the years 1332–1333, another case of leprosy had to be checked. To do so, the Bishop of Lincoln appointed three commissioners, one papal legate, one canon and one professor in civil law to judge whether Richard of Wallingford, Abbot of Saint Alban,[21] had leprosy or not. Unlike Honorius III, John XXII did not request a physician. The medical issue was diagnosed and dealt with by non-medical specialists, which perhaps strengthened the moral dimension of the disease. During the commissioners' visit and examination of the abbot, they noted that Richard had been afflicted with leprosy for five years,

---

[17] Picot (2012: 297).

[18] It is important to note that this is because Theobaldus was being elected as archbishop of Rouen at the time that this denunciation was probably made.

[19] Honorius III—Reg. Vat. 11, f. 237: 'idem Thesaurarius infectus esse dicitur morbo lepre, discretioni vestre sub obtestatione divini iudicii firmiter iniungendo, mandamus quatenus inter alia inquirenda circa hunc articulim advocatis medicis fidelibus et in hoc peritis inquisitionem diligentissimam faciatis'.

[20] Honorius III—Reg. Vat. 11, f. 239.

[21] For two years Abbot Richard had suffered from a progressing case of blindness in his left eye. Thus, it is doubtful that he actually suffered from leprosy. Further, identifying Richard as a leper was the means for his enemy to depose him. Nevertheless, the dispensation letters and St Alban's chronicle use the term *leprosy*—reflecting the fact that his contemporaries most likely classified him as such. In this context, I consider Richard as 'leprous'. On this, see North (1976: 7).

according to the *Chroniques* of St Alban's monastery.[22] The investigators also had to enquire about the damage caused by Richard's infirmity to the monastery more generally, as a result of the abbot's incapacity to govern properly. Another dispensation letter on this case, written by John XXII two months later, on 15 July 1333, stresses the negative spiritual and earthly consequences of the abbot's disease for those around him: "Furthermore, stained by leprous disease caused by divine judgment, [Richard] can not live among healthy people without scandal, so that the whole administration, both for spiritual and temporal matters, is known to be being carried out by means of others."[23]

Similarly, John XXII wrote to the bishop of Autun in a letter dated 22 September 1329 to enquire if he could, personally, inform him as to the (suspected) leprosy of Guidonus, Abbot of Flavigny.[24] From studying dispensation letters, it is clear that popes frequently required investigations in order to confirm—or deny—suspicions of leprosy before making any irreversible decisions as to the cleric's unsuitability. Moreover, in the papal dispensation letters, the popes routinely added a forfeiting clause for the attention of the addressees. Using the words *si est ita* (if that is), the popes signalled that their decisions would be valid only if *lepra* was definitively diagnosed by the direct superiors of the 'leprous' clerics.[25] The fact that the direct superior of a suspected leper-cleric had to check if the cleric really had leprosy reveals the papal willingness to control all clergy levels.

The Disabled Cleric: Between Physical Incapacity and Suitable Representation

In a discussion of the Eucharist, the *Summa Theologica* of Thomas Aquinas maintains that a cleric with a physical deficiency cannot celebrate mass. The disabled cleric cannot save souls and provide the laity with the sacraments because of his infirmity: 'sometimes by making it impossible to exercise them, as, for example, if he lost his

---

[22] Walsingham (1867: 286). See also John XXII—*Regesta,* Vol. 117, f. 116: 'magister Johannes de Offorde, de quo supra scripsimus, decanus de Arcubus, et magister Robertus de Bromlee, officialis magistri Icherii de Contoreto, nuncii Domini Papae, cum commissione eis facta per Episcopum Lincolniensem, ad inquirendum de statu Abbatis et Monasterii; qui suggestum fuit, ut duximus, Domino Papae, quos Abbas fuit jam per quinque annos tam gravi leprae morbo respersus'.

[23] John XXII—Reg. Vat. 105, ep. 1503: 'Adeo est divino iudicio lepre morbo respersus, quod nequit inter sanos absque scandalo conversari propter quod tota administratio ipsius monasteri tam in spiritualibus quod in temporalibus per alios dumtaxat dinoscitur exerceri'.

[24] John XXII—Reg. Vat. 93, ep. 22: 'de huius ipsius abbatis infirmitate per te ipsim diligentius te informes et quecumque super hiis inveneris nobis fideliter per tuas litteras studeas intimare'.

[25] For example, Gregory IX—Reg. Vat. 17, f. 23 r°, or Alexander IV—Reg. Vat. 24, f. 205.

sight, or his fingers, or the use of speech; and sometimes on account of danger, as in the case of one suffering from epilepsy, or indeed any disease of the mind'. Thomas adds that, on occasion, the leper-cleric could provoke such horror in those around him that it would prevent the cleric's exercise of typical duties. This is the case, for example, for a leprous cleric 'who ought not to celebrate in public: he can, however, say mass privately, unless the leprosy has gone so far that it has rendered him incapable owing to the wasting away of his limbs'.[26] This interdiction against public celebration is designed to prevent an incapacity de facto caused by the inability to perform a task required of the clergy. Moreover, the prohibition is also founded upon public contempt for the disease and the desire of the Church to avoid potential scandal. Here, Aquinas utilises leprosy as the most vivid example of a disease that would provoke horror in a clerical sufferer's parishioners; leprosy is the worst disease for a cleric to contract.

Leprosy's power to generate horror is not just due to the concept of the disease as a sign of moral corruption. Indeed, the illness causes genuine disabilities, such as loss of limbs due to its progression or the need for amputations to forestall its spreading ever further. Much more than the cleric's perfect bodies, the idea questioned in the texts discussed above is the fundamental ability of the priest to perform his task. The first canonical texts, such as the *Apostolic Constitutions* dated from AD 375 to 380 and its most famous chapter 47 (*Canons of the Apostles*), allowed a cleric to become a bishop if he was worthy of the episcopal dignity, even if he was 'maimed in an eye (blind), or lame of his leg'. But, this chapter also stresses that a blind or mute man cannot be a bishop. This is to avoid the disruption of ecclesiastical affairs, both spiritual and temporal, for mass or sacraments and management of property law. The canon states that a man could not be a bishop in this case, 'not as being a defiled person, but that the ecclesiastical affairs may not be hindered'.[27] According to that canonical statement, blemishes and injuries of the body were not obstacles to holy orders if the soul was clear from any impurity.

Guidonus, abbot of the monastery of Flavigny founded by the kings of France, under the influence of Philip VI of France and Joan the Lame, was suspected by the latter to be a leper. Indeed, Guidonus was totally incapable of managing and governing his monastery because he lost his tongue (he had some difficulties of speech due to leprosy) and he was 'tarnished' (*respersus*) by *lepra*. This is why the king and queen of France ask the pope to take care of this case before the spiritual and temporal damage to the monastery become permanent: "Our dear son Guidonus, abbot of the monastery [of Flavigny], is totally unsuitable (*inhabilis*) to govern the said monastery, because he lost the benefice of his tongue and he

---

[26] Thomas Aquinas, 1888–1889, III, Q. 82, art. 10, Reply 3.
[27] Coxe, Roberts and Donaldson (1886), VIII, 47.77–47.78.

is splashed by leprosy. So, he can not serve or govern his monastery in spiritual or temporal matters. The king and queen of France implore us to take care with diligence of the spiritual and temporal damage of this monastery."[28]

The loss of speech put Guidonus in a position of ecclesiastical irregularity, specifically as a cleric suffering from the canonical notion of incapacity (*impedimenta*). From the perspective of canon law, total incapacity of the sort experienced by Guidonus precludes an individual from being a member of the clergy, whilst partial incapacity just reduced his sphere of action.[29] Leprosy could make the clerics *inhabiles* (incompetent: fully incapacitated) or *inutiles* (useless: partially incapacitated) to govern their ecclesiastical office.[30]

Leprosy causes incapacity due to its inherent disabling effects. Thus, as a consequence of his disease, the leper-cleric enters into irregularity, which is etymologically derived from the term '*regula*', or rule, which is imposed on all clergy. All irregular clerics were sources of scandal because they publically deviated from the ecclesiastical norm.[31] According to Arnaud Fossier, the Church's fear of scandal reflects an institutional fear of evil as *contagio*. It also shows that a key part of the cleric's role was to be a public *exemplum*. In cases of irregularity, the cleric's capacity and legitimacy as a model could come into question. The Church tried to maintain the clerics' 'orderliness', because clerical indiscipline, if made public, could cause the laity to question their faith and the legitimacy of Church control. The *Decretals of Gregory IX* refer to a letter composed by Clement III which details the necessity of removing a leprous priest from the administration of his office in order to suppress potential scandal and the inevitable contempt of the general public: "The priest who is tarnished by the disease of leprosy because of divine judgment has to be removed from the administration of his office of a parish church because of the scandal and abomination among the people he could provoke."[32]

---

[28] John XXII—Reg. Vat. 93, ep. 22: 'Dilectus filius Guidonis, abbas dicti monasterii, totaliter est factus inhabilis ad regimen et gubernationem ipsius, ex eo quod divino iudicio beneficium linguae perdidit et est etiam lepre morbo respersus, propter quod nequit in spiritualibus et temporalibus ipsius monasteri ministrare sive administratores alii sunt positi in eodem. Quare praefati Rex et Regina nobis humiliter supplicarunt ut ne propter hoc praedictum monasterium in eisdem spiritualibus et temporalibus subeat detrimentum eidem monasterio, in hac parte prospicere paterna diligentia curaremus'.

[29] Naz (1935: VI, 43).

[30] Another example in Clement VI—Reg. Vat. 151, f. 31R: 'cum infirmantibus infirmemur et cum illis maxime qui divino percussi iudicio sibi inutiles et ad aliis contemptibiles reputantur'.

[31] Fossier (2009: 328).

[32] Richter and Friedberg (1881: III–VI, IV): 'De sacerdote vero, qui divino iudicio leprae morbo repercussus in parochiali ecclesia praelationis officio fungitur, dicimus, quod pro

Sometimes, mere suspicion of leprosy in a clergyman was enough to provoke scandal. Thus, the pope wanted to anticipate or avoid scandal and might hide the cleric's *defectus* through the mechanism of papal grace.[33] Returning to the case of Abbot Richard of Wallingforth, after a thorough examination, the investigators declared that Richard could not live with the healthy without provoking *scandalus*. Furthermore, they proclaimed that the abbot could not be a member of the chapter or the chancel with the other brothers, reiterating the pope's earlier statement in his letter. According to the commissioners' diagnosis, the *Chronicle* relates that "This abbot, who was gravely tarnished by leprosy, can not speak with other people without scandal or enter in the monastic chapter or the choir of the church with his monk brothers."[34]

The investigators even predicted the ruin of the monastery if the abbot did not abdicate. Although Richard refused, he could not manage the monastery without assistance. To resolve this problem, he later appointed himself a coadjutor according to the *Chroniques*. In a letter sent a few months later (not recorded in the *Chroniques*), the pope claimed that the bishop threatened witnesses and thus stopped them from giving true testimony about Richard's leprosy.[35]

This is an example of a scandal that motivated papal intervention and the use of dispensation letters in order to control the flow of information to the public and to settle the cleric's discipline. The Church used the category of 'irregularity' to contravene canonical precepts, and ultimately to render the 'irregularity' nullified by authorising it with dispensation letters. In addition, the only way for the pope to interfere in order to prevent scandal was to provoke the ostracism of the cleric. This ostracism could be professional or spatial—or both—leading to social exclusion. We can assume that the pope did so because of the fear of *contagio* (which could be literal or moral, i.e., disease or evil), but also to promote physical perfection and so to avoid the horror that the leper provoked in others.

Professional and Spatial Ostracism Leading to Relative Social Inclusion

The *Decretals of Gregory IX* state that if the rector of a church is leprous, he must be removed from his administrative role. However, the Church had to support such

---

scandalo et abominatione populi ab administrationis debet officio removeri'.
[33] Fossier (2009: 345).
[34] Walsingham (1867: 286); John XXII—*Regesta,* Vol. 117, f. 116: 'Quos Abbas fuit jam per quinque annos tam gravi leprae morbo respersus, quod non posset sine scandalo cum hominibus conversari, neque capitulum aut chorum ingredi inter fratres'.
[35] John XXII—Reg. Vat. 104, f. 477 R: 'Testes autem qui fuerunt nominati si se gracia, odio vel timore subtraxerint censuram simili appellatione cessante compellas veritati testimonium prohibere'.

an individual, including feeding him as much as his church could,³⁶ paying out on a kind of ecclesiastical health insurance. No leprous ex-priest was neglected by the papacy, which took seriously its obligation to take care of all members. Obviously, the sick cleric could not stay in the same position as before. For example, Gregory IX pointed out that, afflicted with *lepra*, a priest of Saint Solen and vicar of Pludishie (in the diocese of Dol) in 1233 could not serve his church anymore without putting his soul in danger, deceiving his parishioners, and spiritually damaging his parish and his vicariate. Although he could not be a priest any longer, he could nevertheless keep his payment owed to the curate or priest, but he had to appoint a vicar to his vicariate who could collate the earning and ensure the administrative or practical functions in the Church, such as the celebration of mass: "R. of Saint Solen, priest in [the recipient (bishop of Dol)]'s diocese, suffers from leprosy and cannot serve his church nor his perpetual vicar of Pludishie, in the Dol diocese because of the danger for his soul and for his church. We allow him a grant of thirty livres Turon, recovered from the dime of his church and other ecclesiastical incomes in order to live conveniently. We also ask that a suitable people is entrusted to serve in his vicariate."³⁷

Nevertheless, the practical work of tending to the spiritual needs of the laity had to be done, so the leprous cleric or his superiors had to appoint a suitable (*idoneus*) assistant to help him. The coadjutor had to ensure the public representation of a *cura animarum* instead of the leper and to share the income with him. The *Decretals of Gregory IX* declared that a rector of a church who is a leper or infected in another way cannot ensure the service of the altar because of the major scandal he could provoke for the healthy people who come to the church. To prevent that, the pope wants an infected rector to have a coadjutor who can manage the *cura animarum* and who can receive a portion of the resources of the Church to sustain him.³⁸ In a French translation of this decretal in an

---

³⁶ Richter and Friedberg (1881: III–VI), Chapter IV.
³⁷ Gregory IX—Reg. Vat. 17, f. 23 r°: 'R. de Sancto Sollemni, presbyterum sue diocese, lepre morbo laboret et propter hoc alicui ecclesie nequeant deservire, nichilominus tamen perpetuam vicariam in ecclesia de Pludishie., Dolensis dioecesis detinere presumit in anime sue periculum et eiusdem ecclesie detrimentum. [. . .] in decimus eiusdem ecclesie et aliis proventibus ecclesiasticis in sua diocese ultra valentiam triginta librarum Turonensis monete unde potest comode sustentari, super hoc providere paterna sollicitudine dignaremur. [. . .] Vicariam ipsam per illos ad quos eius collatio pertinet idonee facias conferri persone qui in eadem ecclesia velit et valeat deservire'.
³⁸ Richter and Friedberg (1881: III–VI), Chapter III (Lucius III): 'De rectoribus ecclesiarum leprae macula usque adeo infectis, quod altari servire non possunt, nec sine magno scandalo eorum, qui sani sunt, ecclesias ingredi, hoc volumus te tenere, quod eis dandus est coadiutor, qui curam habeat animarum, et de facultatibus ecclesiae ad sustentationem suam congruam

anonymous manuscript dating from the mid-12th century, we read that a 'priest with a benefice who becomes a leper can sing without scandal. We ask that he have a coadjutor to take care of the souls'.[39] The translation of this anonymous French author implies that the coadjutor ensured the proper care of souls whilst the priest could no longer sing (perform) mass, a situation stated in the *Decretals of Gregory IX* because the coadjutor had received an earning sufficient to sustain him. Similarly, in the regular clergy, the pope asked the superiors to send to the diseased an administrator to manage the monastery for him.[40] This coadjutor was often chosen from the diseased abbot's circle thanks to his knowledge of the specific monastery.[41]

The scenarios outlined above situate leper-clerics as burdens, completely useless to their churches. They kept their honorific title, but their responsibilities were insignificant and they were, in fact, jobless. Furthermore, their career plans were annihilated by such a relegation from active clerical duties. For example, a friar minor in 1392 was, because of his leprosy, segregated (*segregatus*) from the common fellowship (*consortio*) of his order. He was left as a beggar without any means of subsistence and was turned out of his monastery. The pope allowed him to hold an ecclesiastical office without cure (*simplex*), or a poor hospital, or a hermitage, again with no cure of souls, but at least with an earning.[42]

The spatial isolation experienced by leprous clerics was directly linked to their physical condition. Roger, a priest and rector who was struck by *lepra* in 1256, was allowed by the pope to have a pension. But Alexander IV, in a letter written 23 October 1256 to the archbishop of Rouen, also forced Roger to live in complete isolation, staying in his house without any other resident a stone's throw away.[43]

---

recipiat portionem'.

[39] Godefroy (1881–1902): 'pretre qui avoit benefice devint mesel (leprous), ensi quil ne peut chanter sans scandal. On demande quendist droit on dist quil doit avoir coadjuteur qui ait le cure des ames'.

[40] John XXII—Reg. Vat. 93, ep. 22, refers to the previous quotation.

[41] For example, Richard, the abbot of St Alban, appointed as coadjutor Nicolas of Flamstede, who had been a monk in this institution for some 30 years.

[42] Boniface IX—Reg. Lat. 28, f. 118: 'Tu propter lepram qua in asseris domino permitte percusses a communi ordinis fratres minorum professorum consortio segregatus existat tuque non habeas unde vitam tuam valeas sustentare nec dicti tui ordinis cui victimi et alia necessaria prestat voluntaria et merita mendicitas conditio suddiciat secundum persone tue decentiam iuxta huiusmodi morbi qui opinione homine incurabilis est expressas facere oportunas. [. . .] inclinati tecum ut beneficium ecclesiasticum etiam si simplex officium aut hospitale pauperum seu hermitagium quandoque per clericos quandumque vero per laicos solitum gubernari existat'.

[43] Alexander IV—Reg. Vat. 24, f. 205: 'Ex parte Rogerii, [. . .] fuit propositum coram nobis

This precaution, according to the pope, prevented Roger from causing scandal. In this case, the leper was authorised to stay in his own isolated home because it met the criteria for sequestration far enough away from the healthy.

The rules surrounding the isolation of lepers within monastic communities make the necessity of spatial ostracism even more clear. In the Dominican rule, the leprous monk could not live with other monks, but had to be within the precincts of his monastery, in an isolated place.[44] Yet, if the monastery could not provide this accommodation for a legitimate reason (for example, if there was no space for the leprous isolation), the leprous brother could be transferred to another monastery.[45] There are no records of any papal letters that concern this part of Dominican rule. However, one petition written in 1349 about William Volandi—sub-prior of the Cistercian Order, appointed at the monastery of Sainte Marie des Roches, in the diocese of Auxerre—sheds light on this issue. William lost his benefice of sub-prior because of his bodily default (*defectum corporis*) of leprosy and its consequences. He was then made the beneficiary of revenues from an outbuilding of his monastery, worth 20 livres, in line with the wishes of his prior.[46] The abbot and his assembly sent a request to the pope. The words of the final sentence, which contain the decision made by the chancery, allowed William's superiors to put him in a private house separated from the monastery, even if this contravened the order's and the monastery's constitutions. The pope perhaps overruled the Cistercians with the ultimate aim of standardising the monastic *regulae* under pragmatic principles which already existed in the Dominican rule.

Isolation could be brutal for a cleric; leaving his monastery could be very traumatic and could lead to ostracism. But petitions also show that some leper-

---

quod ipso occulto dei iudicio morbo leprae percusso [. . .] Reliques ecclesie predicta redditibus per sustentatione sua eidem R. reservatis et concessa eidem Rogero morandi quo adiuxerit in quadam domo et ecclesie prefate quam ipsem construxit distante ab ea ut dicitur <u>per iactum lapidis dummodo sine habitantium</u> inibi scandalo possit fieri facultatem'.

[44] The Dominican rule and the book of Dominican constitutions were written at the foundation of the Order. This idea is in both the rule from 1256 and the constitutions from 1375. See also Montford (2002: 98).

[45] Galbraith (1925: 211).

[46] Clement VI—Reg. Suppl. 17, f. 201 R: 'Guillermus Volandi de Brionone [. . .] qui casualiter sicut Deo placuit de infirmitate lepre incurreret et ut asseritur paciatur de punti qui propter hujusmodi <u>defectum</u> per abbatem dicti monasteri et conventu de Ruppibus de dicto monasterio et officio subprioratus eiectus quatenus more pii prioris graciam facientes eidem specialem de Grangia Rubea dicto monasterio de Ruppibus dependent cujus fructus redditus et proventus XX librum parisiensis valorem annum non excedunt [. . .]. Compellatur abbas et conventus facere sibi aliquam domum propre monasterio separatam tamen a conversatione aliarum ubi provideatur sibi de neccessariis'.

clerics chose to leave their monastic communities. The leper Johanes of Pedo asked the pope for permission to reside in the Saint Lazar *leprosarium* in Beziers, a place where he could suffer the creator's flagellation with patience.[47] We can assume that he chose to join a leper colony to avoid public scandal. We can also assume that some clerics preferred exclusion from society in the form of joining a community of other lepers, rather than the experience of exclusion from the Church which would leave them alone, fully isolated. In certain cases, the *leprosarium* offered a social link with which a partial integration in the orders could not compete. For example, in Dover's leper house, sufferers were even tonsured like monks.[48] In another letter written by Clement VI, the leprous cleric Robert of Bours was authorised to enter a leper colony because of his disability. Moreover, he was allowed to choose which location he entered, to be sure that he could stay with his wife,[49] who would dedicate herself to the hospital to take care of the sick.[50]

Conclusion

Supplication and dispensation letters show the complex interconnection of denunciation, judgement and scandalised public opinion in diagnoses and management of clerical leprosy. But, there was not only secular judgement to consider; God is often present in these documents. In the papal letters, leper-clerics seem to be seen in a negative light in every instance. In a letter issued by Clement IV, dated between 15 February 1265 and 23 April 1266, an equivalence is made between leprosy and a bad action inflicting *mala fama* on a man who was at the same time accused of being a leper and of committing the vices of fornication and adultery. By these prosecutions, Clement drew a direct parallel between leprosy and the consequence of God's anger because the leper misbehaved before.[51]

---

[47] Clement VI—Reg. Suppl. 6, f. 341 R: 'John mansionem in domino sancti lazarii sibi civites Bitericensis misericorditer impendendo ut ibidem verbera suum creator pati valeat patienter'.

[48] Rawcliffe (2006: 303).

[49] He was probably married because he was in the minor order.

[50] Clement VI—Reg. Vat. 151, f. 30R: 'Cum dilectus filius Robertus de Bours, dictus Peuboin, clericus coniugatus Morinensis diocese sit morbo lepre percussus et ob hoc dilecta in christo filia Margareta Vailly eius uxor ad eius consorcio separari et in hospitali pauperum Beate Marie Remensis in quo fratres et sorores existunt cupiat in infirmis et pauperibus domino famulari [. . .] Margaretam in eodem hospitali ad servicium infirmorum et pauperum recipi faciatis in sociam et sororem sibique iuxta ipsius hospitalis consuetudinem habitum exhiberi'.

[51] Clement IV—Reg. Vat. 29 A, n° 191: 'propter quod venit in filios diffidentie ira Dei, adiciens quod ejusdem vitii occasione perpetuo a choro predicte Parisiensis ecclesie dicebatur

The majority of papal letters analysed in the course of my research quote God's judgement as a justification that leprosy afflicts some people and not others; this explanation also was typically expressed in contemporary literature.[52] By restating the divine roots of leprosy, the popes did not give any personal opinion on the malady. God let it happen; the deity permitted a disease which was, *opinione homini*, incurable.[53] It is noteworthy that neither of the two petitions discussed in this article resorts to such framing. The first does not mention God at all; the second supplicant writes about chance rather than judgement, probably to clear himself of any charge of moral corruption due to the malady.[54] This notion of fortuity (or occasionalism) is entirely absent from the papal letters, which were probably influenced by hagiographical literature and preferred to spread the idea of God's judgement. Regarding such differences between the letters and the petitions, we can assume that the feelings of others (fear of contagion, for example) were important, even shaping the opinion that lepers had about their own disease. They were afraid of what others might think about their disease, which could be perceived as a malediction or a blessing. This demonstrates the incredible power of the belief that lepers were the subject of God's judgement, positively or negatively, a belief which marked leprosy as different from all other diseases, even in the papal dispensation process. Moreover, these letters offer an insight in the construction of what we may call today 'disability'. Indeed, coupled together, unsuitable representation and physical inability caused social consequences for the ecclesiastical office holder. This last, by means of dispensation papal letters, acquired a new social status, not really as a cleric, neither as a layman. Thus, because of the *defectus corporis* he suffered, the cleric entered in a new category of the canon law where he was socially included in a completely different way.

Bibliography

Aquinas, T. 1888–1889. *Opera omnia iussu impensaque Leonis XIII P. M. edita, Summae theologiae*. Rome: Ex Typographia Polyglotta S. C. de Propaganda Fide.

Aquinas, T., Busa, R., Bernot, E., and Alarcón, E. 2005. *Index thomisticus*. Navarre: Fundación Tomás de Aquino.

---

ejectus, quodque de morbo lepre suspectus erat, et de fornicatione vel adulterio procreatus necnon inhoneste conversationis ac perjurii crimine irretitus existens, Parisius errores pluries predicavit'. On the association of a disease to different sins, see, for example, Stearns (2011: 52 or 169).

[52] On the 13 letters I use for this study, 11 quoted God's judgment.
[53] Boniface IX—Reg. Lat. 28, f. 118. See quotation above.
[54] Clement VI—Reg. Suppl. 6, f. 341 R, by the words 'morbo lepre percussit'; or in Clement VI—Reg. Suppl. 17, f. 201 R: 'casualiter sicut Deo placuit de infirmitate lepre incurreret'.

Bériac, F. 1990. *Des lépreux aux cagots: recherches sur les sociétés marginales en Aquitaine médiévale.* Bordeaux: Fédération historique du Sud-Ouest, Institut d'histoire, Université de Bordeaux III.

Bériou, N. and Touati, F. -O. 1991. *Voluntate dei leprosus: les lépreux entre conversion et exclusion aux XIIème et XIIIème siècles.* Spoleto: Centro Italiano di studi Sull'altro Medioevo.

Catholic Church, Cancellaria Apostolica and Archivio Segreto Vaticano, 1198. *Registra Vaticana.*

Catholic Church, Cancellaria Apostolica and A.S.V., 1389. *Registra lateranensia.*

Catholic Church, Dataria Apostolica and A.S.V., 1342. *Registra supplicationum.*

Covey, H. C. 2001. People with Leprosy (Hansen's Disease) During the Middle Ages. *Social Science Journal* 38(2): 315–321.

Coxe, A. C., Roberts, R. A., Donaldson, J. (eds) 1886. *The Ante-Nicene Fathers: translations of the writings of the Fathers down to A.D. 325*, vol. 7. Buffalo (NY): Apostolic Teaching and Constitutions, Christian Literature Co.

Demaitre, L. E. 2007. *Leprosy in Premodern Medicine: A Malady of the Whole Body.* Baltimore: Johns Hopkins University Press.

Fossier, A. 2009. Propter vitandum scandalum. Histoire d'une catégorie juridique (XIIe–XVe siècles). *Mélanges de l'Ecole Française de Rome Moyen Âge* 121: 317–348.

Galbraith, G. R. 1925. *The Constitution of the Dominican Order, 1216-1360.* Manchester: The University Press.

Godefroy, F. 1881–1902. *Dictionnaire de l'ancienne langue française et de tous ses dialectes du IXe au XVe siècle.* Paris: F. Vieweg.

Guaydier, G. 1933. *Les irrégularités 'ex defectu corporis': Thèse présentée pour le doctorat en droit canonique.* Paris: Société Générale d'Imprimerie et d'Edition.

Hays, J. 2009. *The Burdens of Disease Epidemics and Human Response in Western History,* revised ed. Piscataway (NJ): Rutgers University Press.

Hermann, C. 2009. *Lépreux et maladières dans l'ancien diocèse de Genève du XIIIe siècle au début du XVIe siècle.* Chambéry: Société savoisienne d'histoire et d'archéologie.

Jeanne, D. 2014. Leprosy, Lepers and Leper-Houses: Between Human Law and God's Law (6th–15th centuries, in S. Crawford and C. Lee (eds), *Social Dimensions of Medieval Disease and Disability,* Studies in Early Medicine 3: 69–82. Oxford: Archaeopress.

Löfstedt, L. 1993. *Gratiani decretum 2, Causae 1-14.* Soc. Scient. Helsinki: Fennica.

Mansi, J. D. 1961. *Sacrorum conciliorum nova et amplissima collectio,* vol. 22, Graz: Akad. Dr.- u. Verl.-Anst.

Marcombe, D. 2003. *Leper Knights the Order of St Lazarus of Jerusalem in England, c. 1150-1544.* Woodbridge: Boydell Press.

Merzbacher, F. 1967. Die Leprosen im alten kanonischen Recht. *Zeitschrift der Savigny-Stiftung für Rechtsgeschichte. Kanonistische Abteilung* 53(1): 27–45.

Miller, T. S. and Nesbitt, J. W. 2014. *Walking Corpses Leprosy in Byzantium and the Medieval West.* Ithaca (NY): Cornell University Press.

Montford, A. 2002. Fit to Preach and Pray: Considerations of Occupational Health in the Mendicant Orders, in R. N. Swanson (ed.), *The Use and Abuse of Time in Christian History:* 95–106. Woodbridge: Boydell Press.

Naz, R. 1935. *Dictionnaire de droit canonique.* Paris: Letouzey et Ané.

Noble, T., Wycliffe, J, and Purvey, J. 2010. *Wycliffe's Old Testament Translated by John Wycliffe and John Purvey: A Modern-Spelling Edition of Their 14th Century Middle English Translation.* Vancouver: Terry Noble.

North, J. D. 1976. *Richard of Wallingford: An Edition of His Writings.* Oxford: Clarendon Press.

Picot, J. 2012. 'La Purge': une expertise juridico-médicale de la lèpre en Auvergne au Moyen Âge. *Revue Historique* 662: 292–321.

Rawcliffe, C. 2006. *Leprosy in Medieval England.* Woodbridge: Boydell Press.

Richter, E. L. and Friedberg, E. (eds) 1879. *Corpus Iuris Canonici, Decretum magistri Gratiani.* Leipzig: Bernahrd Tauchnitz.

Richter, E. L. and Friedberg, E. (eds) 1881. *Corpus Iuris Canonici, Pars Secunda, Decretalium Collectiones Decretales Gregorii p. IX.* Leipzig: Bernahrd Tauchnitz.

Stearns, J. K. 2011. *Infectious Ideas: Contagion in Premodern Islamic and Christian Thought in the Western Mediterranean.* Baltimore: Johns Hopkins University Press.

Tabuteau, B. 2012. Vingt mille léproseries au Moyen Âge? Tradition française d'un poncif historiographique. *Memini. Travaux et documents* 15: 115–124.

Touati, F. -O. 1998. *Maladie et société au Moyen Age: la lèpre, les lépreux et les léproseries dans la province ecclésiastique de Sens jusqu'au milieu du XIVe siècle.* Brussels: De Boeck University.

Touati, F. -O. 2000. Contagion and Leprosy: Myth, Ideas and Evolution in Medieval Minds and Societies, in L. I. Conrad and D. Wujastyk (eds), *Contagion: Perspectives from Pre-modern Societies*: 179–201. Burlington (VT): Ashgate.

Walsingham, T. 1867. *Chronica monasterii S. Albani, Gesta abbatum monasterii Sancti Albani, a Thoma Walsingham, regnante Ricardo Secundo, ejusdem ecclesia praecentore, compilata. 2. A. D. 1290-1349.* London: Henry Thomas Riley Reader.

Weber, R., Gryson, R., and Fischer, B. 2007. *Biblia sacra: iuxta Vulgatam versionem.* Stuttgart: Deutsche Bibelgesellschaft.

Winroth, A. 2004. *The Making of Gratian's Decretum.* New York: Cambridge University Press.

Wycliffe, J. and Purvey, J. 2012. *Bible* 1395. Terence P. Noble (ed.), Vancouver: Terence P. Noble.

Acknowledgements

I thank Alicia Spencer-Hall, for the amazing help she provided to write this paper, and the editors, Stefanie Künzel and Erin Connelly, for their kind remarks.

Inside the *Leprosarium*: Illness in the Daily Life of 14th-Century Barcelona

Clara Jáuregui

The present work is a first glance at one of the richest sources we have about the *leprosarium* of Barcelona: its account books. Although they comprise a short period of time (1379–1395), these books give valuable information of all kinds: economic, religious, medical, alimentary, social, etc. This paper aims to increase our knowledge of a hospital that has been ignored, providing new data from these books that until now have not been studied. This hospital has been overlooked possibly because the sources were not known or perhaps because it was assumed that the history of the *leprosarium* was already written. Fortunately, the voices of the past can still enlighten us today.

Previous Studies and Perspectives

At this point, there is only one published paper, authored by Aurora Pérez Santamaría, focusing in depth on the Hospital of Saint Margaret (also called Saint Lazarus, depending on the century). For many years, her work has been crucial to understanding how and when the *leprosarium* of Barcelona appeared.[1] But her study of the sources found in the diocesan and cathedral's archives was, probably due to lack of time, incomplete in a number of ways. The subsequent works of Anna Castellano and James Brodman tried to broaden her previous study. They focused mainly on donations, sale deeds and episcopal ordinances.[2] However, some of these documents, such as the account books, remained untouched, even though the range of information in them is wider than the rest of the sources.[3] Few other studies have focused on the architecture, the art and the archaeological remains of the hospital.[4] Despite this variety, and given the fact that most of them repeated

---

[1] Pérez Santamaría (1980: 75–116).
[2] Castellano (1994: 41–50); Brodman (1998: 35–45).
[3] Pérez Santamaría presents a general overview of the account book from 1379 to 1381, which is focused on economic data. However, the account overlooks important data relative to the patients and the daily life of the place.
[4] *Lambard: Estudis d'art medieval* (1994) has different papers focused on these subjects.

Pérez Santamaría's work, a big picture does not present itself when looking at the *leprosarium* as a whole.

Moreover, the first study about this institution, from the 19th century, has to be revisited in light of new approaches formulated in the past few years, which changed scholarly opinions about lepers and their exclusion.[5] Ideas like segregation or the ritual of civil death cannot be upheld when confronted with the sources at hand.[6] There is, for instance, no direct or indirect reference in the account books to any ceremony performed when a new patient arrived at this hospital. The present study of this new source fills an important gap on how this institution was managed and how the patients lived there.

Sources

As mentioned before, Pérez Santamaría began the study of some remaining account books held at the cathedral's archive from the period of 1379–1395. However, she focused mainly on the first of eight volumes.[7] Also, Brodman used her information to extrapolate this partial data and describe the daily life at this hospital. The books, written by the different managers of the hospital, are a window into the lives of not only the managers, but also the patients and workers. All of them follow the same pattern of division by incoming register, exit register and daily expenses.[8] Each book counts the money of two whole years, making notes daily of the donations received at the church, at one of the altars of the cathedral, the sale of bread, the expenses and benefits of the orchard, the food and medicine purchased, and the arrivals and deaths of patients. Written in Catalan and excellently well preserved, they are similar to a journal in their description of the events that affected life at the hospital, including major events in the larger history of the city such as the attacks on the Jewish Quarter in 1391. The information provided about the daily events is always brief but very descriptive, giving us new data on the building, its properties, its workers and, more importantly, the patients. For example, 'costs the

---

[5] Brenner (2010); Rawcliffe (2006); De Maitre (2007).
[6] Brodman (1998: 42).
[7] Arxiu Capitular de Barcelona (ACB), Hospital de Santa Margarida, Llibres de comptes, 1379–1395. One of them is actually misclassified and belongs to another hospital. It needs to be clarified that the paper of Aurora Pérez Santamaría was based on her BA thesis and, therefore, perhaps due to time constraints, she decided to focus mainly on the Diocesan documentation.
[8] The fact that the books of the other two hospitals (Colom and d'en Vilar) that were under chapter management followed the same pattern seems to imply some type of control of the accounts and inspections. The ordinances studied by Pérez Santamaría also show how at some point the hospital's managers might have been embezzling funds.

bloodletting of two patients 1 *sou*' or 'one mattress for Guillem [a patient]'. Apart from the importance of the books as a source for information about daily life, they might also be a good testimony of the fading of this institution and the sickness itself.

Origins of the Hospital

There are still many gaps in the knowledge about this hospital, especially when it comes to its origins. For many years, the 12th century has been accepted as the foundation date, although there is no documentation to support this. The first to give an estimated date was Josep Maria Roca, who suggested that a bishop called Guillem presumably founded it in the 9th century. The problem is that, like many 19th-century historians, Josep Maria Roca rarely cited his sources. Besides, there is no record of a bishop in the 9th century called Guillem. Therefore, researchers deduced that Josep Maria Roca must have been referencing Bishop Guillem de Torroja, who lived in the 12th century (1144–1174), thus moving the foundation of the hospital to that century without actual proof.[9] A more reliable source is Bishop Ponç de Gualba (14th century). In the ordinances of the hospital that Ponç de Gualba made, he discusses his 'predecessor' Guillem as founder, but only mentions his name.[10] The first documents related to the hospital are donations and sale deeds from the end of the 12th century. It is probable that the creation of a *leprosarium* was around that time, but without more data, we cannot be sure. The extant Romanesque church may be interpreted in support of the 12th-century record, but nothing rules out the possibility that the hospital could have been built before the church.

Barcelona's Hospital Network

In comparison with the other hospitals of Barcelona, the 12th century appears to be the most probable date for the foundation of the *leprosarium*. Ecclesiastical hospitals proliferated in the 12th century, especially those that were linked to monasteries. Until the 13th–14th centuries, secular foundations did not expand Barcelona's hospital network. Perhaps that is why, in the 12th and 13th centuries, the *leprosarium* was called *domus infirmorum ac pauperum* (house for the sick and poor). When there were fewer hospitals available, this one might have been used for lepers and poor people at the same time, as early 14th-century ordinances

---

[9] Pérez Santamaría (1980: 78).
[10] ADB (Arxiu Diocesà de Barcelona), Notularum Communium, 1325–1330, f. 62v–63v.

suggest.[11] With the increase of foundations in the city, there was no need to maintain this situation, and the denomination changed to *hospitalem infirmorum ac leprosorum* (house for the sick and lepers). It is not the only hospital to undergo this process; many other foundations in Catalonia, such as Girona and Lleida, for instance,[12] seem to have followed the same path.

The network appeared fully transformed by 1401, when the six remaining hospitals of the city merged into the General Hospital, which is located very close to the *leprosarium*. This hospital remained at the same site until 1906—although under different management.[13]

Urban Context

The isolated location of the *leprosarium* has been assumed to be a consequence of the social exclusion and rejection of lepers. However, as we will see in the following sections, this might not be the case. In the 12th century, the city grew outside its first Roman wall and there was no space available for such purpose. In 1285, King Pere II ordered the construction of a second wall, which left the *leprosarium* and other hospitals on the outside. This situation is similar to that of Santa Eulàlia del Camp (incidentally, this monastery was founded by Guillem de Torroja in 1155) or the Hospital of Colom (founded in 1219).[14] The *leprosarium* and the Hospital of Colom were located along paths that led to the city gates (the Portal de La Boqueria and Porta Ferrissa)—that is, relatively close to the city. When a third wall was eventually built (1357), these hospitals and a third one (Hospital d'en Vilar, 1311) were enclosed inside it, and the surrounding area was starting to be occupied by the inhabitants of the city. A new city gate, the Portal de Sant Antoni, completed in 1377, led travelers directly to these hospitals. At the end of the 14th century, the presumed isolation would have been practically nonexistent.

Barcelona is not the only city that seems to have a *leprosarium* in its immediate vicinity. Therefore, the theory that these foundations were always isolated should be thoroughly revised if not altogether dismissed. Studies such as Carole Rawcliffe's *Leprosy in Medieval England* have opened new ways of interpreting the location of these institutions.[15] In the Crown of Aragon, the pattern seems to

---

[11] 'Infirmorum ac leprosorum aliorumque pauperum Christi et miserabilium personarum nostre diochesis'. ADB (Arxiu Diocesà de Barcelona), Notularum Communium, 1325–1330, f. 62v–63v.
[12] Guilleré (1980).
[13] Danon (1978).
[14] Lindgren (1980).
[15] Rawcliffe (2006).

follow populated areas or important roads that led to urban hotspots, such as city gates. That is the case, for example, in Monzón, where the *leprosarium* is located near the city wall.[16] The same happens in Catalonia with cities such as Tarragona. Theories that connect the pilgrimage in the Way of St James with the spreading of these institutions, to take care of pilgrims and lepers, do not seem to take into consideration their proximity to villages or cities, fitting the *leprosaria* into a hospital network they do not belong to.[17] With these new perspectives, we can assume that the urban context of these *leprosaria* is critical to their survival.

The House

Today, the church is all that remains of this institution. It is a small Romanesque chapel with altars dedicated to Saint Margaret and Saint Lazarus, the two names the hospital adopted. An archaeological excavation in 1989–1991 verified the past existence of a hospital next to it with a small wooden bridge that connected the two buildings.[18] Although they found burials from different periods inside the church, the remains do not seem to carry any physical markers that might suggest cases of leprosy. A new archaeological study was conducted between 2007 and 2009, and more burials were found outside the church. An osteological study is ongoing, and therefore evidence of leprosy might still be discovered. Among the burials, there are nine simple graves and nine common graves (52 individuals) from the 14th century that seem to belong to the hospital's cemetery.[19] As the other graves inside the church had funerary objects, archaeologists identified them as the graves of the patients. In those mass graves a fair number of children and adolescents are buried, which are not present in the documental sources.[20] There is, however, a brief reference to a common grave used during the 'great mortality from the bygone days', which might explain these finds, linking them to some episode of plague.[21] The cemetery was not excavated in its entirety, and there might be more burials still unexplored. Apart from the burials, the excavations found that between the 14th and the 15th centuries, renovations were undertaken at the hospital, which provided new buildings for the patients. As there is no record of these renovations in the account books (only a roof repair), we may narrow the dating of the newer buildings to the 15th century.

---

[16] Villagrasa (2015: 204).
[17] Lázaro (1994).
[18] López and Beltran de Heredia (1994: 41–71).
[19] Triay Olives (2007–2009: 28).
[20] Triay Olives (2007–2009: 29–31).
[21] ACB, Hospital de Santa Margarida, 1385, f. 12r.

We cannot say for certain how big the hospital was, although the sources give us a pretty good idea of the way it was arranged. Apart from the church, the hospital had a kitchen garden annex that provided not only food, but also a surplus to sell at the market. The hospital itself was composed of a kitchen, a room for the manager, another one for the housekeeper and two rooms for the patients, separated by gender. Possibly, it had other rooms or houses, as the 2007 excavations show, but it is difficult to determine which ones are from the period in question and what purposes they had. From time to time, the account books inform us about maintenance repairs on the rooms and the roof, as well as on how the women's room was closed off for a period of time because there were not any women at the hospital.

What is not clear is if all the workers of the house lived there too or just stayed for their meals. There is a brief note of mattresses for two messengers, so we can deduce that at least some of them stayed there.[22] Around five people worked there daily (apart from the manager, who acted as *hospitaler*), including the messengers, the maids (*macipas*), the housekeeper and the workers of the orchard and vineyards. The workers were on a salary, although they had short contracts and therefore the rotation was frequent.[23] There is no evidence of lay people working there as *donats/donades*, but it does not exclude them. It might be that in this specific period of time, when the influx of patients was lower, the influx of *donats* was also low. Among the workers, we can find special cases, such as the wife of one of the patients, Caterina, who stayed even after the death of her husband.[24] It has been suggested that in the early times of the institution, a religious community, perhaps a monastery, was in charge of the patients, but no evidence has been found to support this.[25] There were also temporary workers in the vineyards and orchards of the hospital. They were employed seasonally, and a whole section of every book details the maintenance and development work, especially in the winemaking process.

The hospital also had a slave, Vicens, who was supposed to help with the work, but, apparently, caused more problems than he solved. The different managers wrote unsparingly of how he was always drunk, fighting with someone (other slaves or lepers of the house), how he was hurt in those fights or how he ended up in prison for hurting someone.[26] Curiously, he was also constantly sick

---

[22] ACB, Hospital de Santa Margarida, Llibres de comptes, 1393–1395, f. 39r.
[23] A housekeeper stayed only 11 days because she said she was not pleased with the house. ACB, Hospital de Santa Margarida, Llibres de comptes, 1383–1385, f. 87r.
[24] ACB, Hospital de Santa Margarida, Llibres de comptes, 1389–1391, f. 89r.
[25] Pérez Santamaría (1980: 90).
[26] ACB, Hospital de Santa Margarida, Llibres de comptes, 1385–1387, f. 93r.

and receiving treatment or a special diet because of it. One of the managers had a particularly difficult confrontation with him after he returned to the *leprosarium* drunk. Vicens threatened to snap his neck and burn down the hospital, which forced the manager to seek help from the neighbours in order to restrain him.[27] The manager explains how this behaviour is not unusual and how he had previously threatened the housekeeper. Although Vicens was admonished, his behaviour did not change. He died in the hospital, and no other slave took his place.

The Neighbours

As stated previously, at the end of the 14th century the *leprosarium* was far from isolated. There were two other hospitals near it, and a whole neighbourhood started to appear in this part of the city. The fight between the slave and one of the managers gives us a sense of how close the *leprosarium* was to those citizens who came to the manager's aid.

    The *leprosarium* not only interacted with that part of the neighbourhood, it was always in contact with the whole city. As an institution, perhaps the most notorious evidence is left in their interactions with other hospitals, as the interactions with citizens are somewhat obscured by anonymity. In the exchanges with other hospitals, the network of the city is exposed and the scarcity of means the *leprosarium* had in general becomes evident. It had to cooperate when resources and space for new patients decreased. The *leprosarium* frequently had patients redirected from the Hospital of the City, even though some of them were not lepers.[28] At least on one occasion a patient was returned to the original hospital because he was not diagnosed with leprosy.[29] Others arrived on the verge of death, and it would seem that they were not diagnosed at all. It seems that the manager had to choose how many people he would be able to help with his scarce means. Indeed, it was a forced and complex cooperation, as the hospitals were equally underfunded.

    Another example of cooperation between hospitals occurred in 1340, when the administrators of the Hospital of Colom and the *domus infirmorum* traded kitchen equipment and bedding. The administrators and *hospitalers* of Santa Eulalia del Camp, the hospital of Pere de Vilar and the hospital of Marcús were also present and confirmed the exchange.[30] This example shows how they were lacking even basic means.

---

[27] ACB, Hospital de Santa Margarida, Llibres de comptes, 1379–1380, f. 52v–53r.
[28] ACB, Hospital de Santa Margarida, Llibres de comptes, 1381–1382, f. 15r, f. 62r.
[29] ACB, Hospital de Santa Margarida, Llibres de comptes, 1385–1387, f. 59v.
[30] ACB, Manuals Notarials, Bernat de Vilarrúbia, vol. 13, f. 91v–92r.

These exchanges were normal between the hospitals of Barcelona, but, probably due to the nature of the sickness, the *leprosarium* did not receive the same flux of patients. The other hospitals mainly had problems with reallocating foundlings. Depending on wet nurses and available funds, small children were often sent to another place, but never to the *leprosarium*.[31]

It was quite common that hospitals run by the same institution (the chapter or the city council) cooperated on a regular basis—perhaps not always in an agreeable manner, but the daily work made it necessary. There must have been some competition for alms, especially among those hospitals situated close together or close to the city gates, but it is difficult to know the impact that the proximity of other hospitals had upon alms and other donations. Many of the cathedral's altars, for example, collected alms for different hospitals, which might suggest that citizens donated equally to them. Wills from this period confirm this also, with all the hospitals recipient of charity.[32]

The Funds and the Management

The funding to maintain such a household came from different places. The main source was the chapter of the cathedral. Officials from the chapter were responsible for providing the weekly income and also visited from time to time in order to keep an eye on the accounts and state of affairs. However, this money was probably not enough to pay for all the expenses, and the inhabitants of the hospital spent most of their day begging for more financial support.

Even the patients were expected to beg in the city, and the money was used partly for themselves and partly for the hospital. Only those who were especially sick were excused from doing so—for example, a woman who could not move from her bed.[33] The patients were not the only ones responsible for seeking money; there were workers at the hospital especially for that purpose. One of the largest sources of income was the gathering of bread donated by citizens and the subsequent selling of the bread to make a profit. To that end, every morning two or three messengers went to beg for bread and afterwards to the market in order to sell it.

The alms at the church and one of the cathedral's altars were also an assured source of income, just like the donations of properties (houses, lands, emphyteutic

---

[31] The reallocating was especially dramatic after the attacks in 1391 on the Jewish Quarter, when new orphans arrived to all hospitals and the city council had to take the matter into their hands (ACB, Llibre de comptes de l'Hospital de Colom, 1391–1392, f. 96r–97v; ACB, Llibre de comptes de l'Hospital d'en Vilar, 1391–1392, f. 61r and f. 96v).

[32] ACB, Bernat de Vilarrúbia, vol. 42 (1300–1339).

[33] ACB, Hospital de Santa Margarida, 1393–1395, f. 59v.

leases, etc.) of former patients and their families. However, not all the properties of the hospital were donations. The hospital had vineyards that could produce wine for the needs of the house and a surplus that could be sold.

After the daily expenses of the hospital were covered, the remaining money was distributed as a weekly pay between the patients and the workers. This pay was supposed to help them maintain themselves, especially with food (*companatge*), and was increased by the chapter when it was deemed necessary—for instance, on special occasions like important festivities.[34] It was also probably a big incentive to those that went to the hospital, an assured income that could have been more attractive than the stay at the place. As we will see later, the mobility of patients was high, and perhaps some of them did not look for a permanent place but rather for help to continue their journey.

Unfortunately, managers are difficult to understand. Even though they talk to us directly in the account books, they say very little about themselves. The exact position they occupied is a bit blurred, as it would seem that they were not *hospitalers*, which was a position used in the Crown of Aragon, where hospital managers and their families closely cared for the patients. It is not clear if they were all clerics, although it the majority seem to have been presbyters.

Patients' Background and Their Mobility

In 1326, Bishop Ponç de Gualba issued some ordinances to control the proper use of the hospital.[35] Among them was a very specific order to take in new patients, depending on their origin, giving priority to those closer to the city. At the end of the 14th century, the origin of the *leprosarium*'s patients is certainly a matter to analyse closely, as many of them were foreigners. The decline of the sickness probably resulted in vacancies for those foreigners who typically would not have found shelter there.

The patients were not the only ones staying at the hospital; sometimes their own families accompanied them. Although it looks like the families stayed for shorter periods, the managers did not reject them or issue complaints about having extra people to provide for. The presence of families raises the issue of the apparent acceptance of couples and sexuality. Although men and women had different chambers, married couples might have had other privileges.[36]

---

[34] For example, during Lent. In one case, the pay was different depending on the origin of the patients. Patients born Christian received more money than others did, such as Martí, a former slave (ACB, Hospital de Santa Margarida, Llibres de comptes, 1393–1395, f. 62r).

[35] Pérez Santamaría (1980: 81–91).

[36] For example, Caterina and Jordi, worker and patient, respectively. See the first section.

The mobility of the patients shown in the account books is certainly higher than one expects of a marginalised group. To begin with, lepers came and went, suggesting that travelling itself was not an issue. They came from as far as Tartary, presumably using transport such as ships or caravans, and sometimes just stayed a short time in Barcelona before resuming their trip.[37] They left without anyone restraining them and no discharge was necessary. The physicians were consulted when a new patient arrived, but never when they left. The managers seem not to have been concerned about this mobility, perhaps because someone leaving was one less person to provide for. That was the case of a certain Barçalona, who left with her son because she was cured (and therefore was not a leper anymore). It was not the only case of healing, as another woman left stating the same.[38] As we saw earlier, the hospital did not have money to sustain a great number of patients, and the main focus of this place seems to have been to provide temporal help more than seclude patients. The duration of their stay was apparently the decision of the patients and not the managers.

Nevertheless, sickness and recovery were not the only motives to travel; there were also pilgrims among the patients. The patients were not pilgrims who stopped at Barcelona to rest, but some of them, while staying at the hospital, decided to go on pilgrimage and then return to this hospital in particular. Some of these were short journeys, like the one to Montserrat, but at least in one case, we can find a woman taking the Way of St James and coming back to the hospital.[39] These pilgrimages were probably in search of a miracle and healing, and the choosing of the holy place may have been subject to the state of the sickness of the patient.

The lepers came from varied origins and occasionally far afield.[40] In the account books, there are documented patients from Tartary, Greece, Germany, Tuscany, Castile and the whole Crown of Aragon. Their names were not always recorded, and sometimes they were adapted into their Catalan form (for example, Andreu Alemany for Andreas German). What we lack, for the most part, is why

---

[37] That is, if they were accepted in such a means of transportation or had the money to pay for it, something that should be discussed.

[38] 'Margoy left because she wanted to; as she said she was not sick.' ACB, Hospital de Santa Margarida, Llibres de comptes, 1383–1385, f. 53v.

[39] ACB, Hospital de Santa Margarida, Llibres de comptes, 1383–1385, f. 76r. Montserrat is a mountain near Barcelona with an important monastery and a black Virgin Mary that has been a center of pilgrimage in Catalonia for centuries. For more information, see Albareda (1931).

[40] Toda, a woman from Tartary, is the only first name recorded from there, but not the only patient coming from that place. ACB, Hospital de Santa Margarida, Llibres de comptes, 1389–1391, f. 61r.

they travelled so far, particularly because most of them seem to have ended their journey in Barcelona. Maybe medieval lepers had the social sense of a vagrant and some of them travelled until their body had enough. That would go against the idea of isolation and regulation often associated with this sickness. Although perhaps sometimes rejected, the lepers were still part of society.

There are also cases where mobility does not have a positive aspect, as in the case of two patients who stole the weekly pay and ran away. Strangely enough, they returned a week later, on St Lazarus Day, and no reprimand was recorded in the books.[41] Therefore, apart from their impunity, their liberty to come and go from the *leprosarium* seems obvious.

Among the patients, there is no record of Jews or Saracens, only of former slaves (therefore, converted). Given the fact that no other hospital in the city sheltered them and that the city had an active Jewish hospital in the 14th century, Jewish patients would have been cared for there in all likelihood.[42]

Daily Life

Every account book has a whole section focused on the daily expenses, similar to a journal, which is the most detailed and useful part, as this is also where the entrance of new patients and expenses associated with them were written down. Sometimes the books look like shopping lists, but important details of the housework and the sickness itself can still be found.

The food purchased was always a complement to the food produced at the hospital, mainly vegetables such as cabbages or pumpkins. Purchases were mainly of meat (fish during Lent), mutton above all, seasonal vegetables or fruits, spices or cheese. Of particular interest is the food distributed to those who were sick (therapeutic food). It did not matter if a person had a cold or was terminally ill, the food given and the procedure followed was the same. In those cases of sickness, there was an increase in the consumption of chicken, mutton, sugar, dried fruits and nuts. Spiced water was also given as a therapeutic drink. If a patient's condition was severe, then a physician was called and medicine provided, but the first treatment was always a special diet.

Every day patients and workers shared a meal, while the rest of the meals were on their weekly money, the *companatge* (literally, something to eat with bread, which was also provided by the hospital). Temporary workers, such as the ones that worked at the vineyard, also had their meals paid for and sometimes ate

---

[41] ACB, Hospital de Santa Margarida, Llibres de comptes, 1387–1389, f. 54v–55r.
[42] ACB, Notaris, Guillem Torell, vol. 90, f. 53v; AHPB, Pere de Pujol, 33/2, 1385, f. 89r.

with the rest of the house. On special festivities or for funerals, a big meal of better quality and quantity was provided.

The *leprosarium* made its own wine and purchased it only when the vintage was apparently spoiled. There were also special occasions when better wine (white or *grech*) was bought for inspectors and members of the chapter who went to the hospital to check on the state of affairs. Despite the budget, the manager purchased little luxuries like this from time to time.

Facing the Illness

The patients were always called *malalts* (sick person) or *mesells*, the vernacular word for leper. Although the word *leprós/lebrós* (in Catalan) also exists, it is rarely used, and when it is used, it is to say that someone is suffering from the illness (*malalt de llebrosia*). Strangely enough, the patients of other hospitals were also called *malalts*, although these hospitals were supposed to be focused on the poor and destitute. This fact may be due to the link in the Middle Ages between poverty and sickness.

Physicians typically made a leprosy diagnosis, while barbers performed the everyday cures, such as bloodlettings. Physicians intervened only when another illness was suspected (such as a cold or cancer),[43] but mostly their work consisted of determining if a condition was leprosy or not.[44] These physicians were paid for their services, although, supposedly since 1337, they were responsible for seeing all the hospital's patients free of charge.[45] These physicians did not visit the patients in order to cure them, but to provide palliative care. Wounds and discomfort were treated and, even though the sickness itself was dismissed as impossible to cure, purges and honey for the wounds were applied. In some cases, the sickness could only be soothed with new and lighter clothes.[46] A barber performed bloodlettings almost weekly. A strange case is that of Martí, who arrived saying he was sick,

---

[43] That was the case of a leper, Alfons, who was said to have cancer in his mouth. ACB, Hospital de Santa Margarida, Llibres de comptes, 1381–1382, f. 65r–v.

[44] The identity of the physician is unknown in most cases, although, from time to time, an extra piece of information is given, such as a first name, or that a female physician (*metgessa*) had treated a patient. ACB, Hospital de Santa Margarida, Llibres de comptes, 1381–1382, f. 120r.

[45] King Pere III ordered this to physicians and surgeons of Barcelona, although a century later the same was asked in places like Lleida (ACA, reg. 862, f. 101, cited at Conejo 2003: 505). The records of the hospitals of Barcelona (in the 14th and 15th centuries) show how physicians were systematically paid for their job, which seems to invalidate this law (ACB, Hospitals, Llibres de comptes de l'Hospital de Colom i d'en Vilar; AHSCSP, Notaris, Llibres de comptes de l'Hospital de la Santa Creu).

[46] ACB, Hospital de Santa Margarida, Llibres de comptes, 1381–1382, f. 117v.

presumably with leprosy. He was then taken to a physician and cured.⁴⁷ The information in the account book is so brief that we cannot be sure if he really was a leper, if he had another sickness and was cured, or, most improbable, if they considered the leprosy to be cured.

The case of Martí is not the only case of someone being cured. Na Barçalona, who stayed for months with her son, started to feel better until she recovered.⁴⁸ Then they realised she was not suffering from leprosy; the cure itself was proof of it. After she was cured, the manager and her son, Joan, talked about some contribution to the hospital to pay for their stay. Na Barçalona and her son did not have a lot of money, but they wanted to pay something out of gratitude for the care. That raises the question of whether she would have paid anything if she were a leper.

On another occasion, the manager preferred to pay a man called Pere from Valencia directly because he was not sure he was sick and, as the manager admits, it would have been more expensive to call a doctor to make a proper diagnosis.⁴⁹ The man was paid to leave, which also raises the question of how many potential patients were dismissed only because of the hospital's lack of funds. This would collide strongly with any purpose of containing the sickness the *leprosarium* had.

This process of diagnosis is illustrated in all its splendour in the case of a German named Andreu. He arrived at the hospital claiming to be a leper, although all those who examined him (two physicians and a barber) said he was not a leper.⁵⁰ The manager, therefore, told him to leave, but he returned afterwards, claiming again that he was a leper and, more importantly, that he wanted to be a leper. The inspectors of the hospital decided to let him stay until he received another diagnosis, which unfortunately is not written in the account books. The impetuosity of Andreu was probably due to the weekly pay and the possibility to beg good money as a leper. There were other hospitals that provided similar care to the poor, but maybe their patients weren't seen as worthy or needy of charity as lepers.

There are cases when the manager allowed someone who was not a leper to stay at the hospital—for example, a woman with a deformed face and hearing and visual impairments.⁵¹ However, as she was able to beg for money, he did not give her an allowance. The doors were open for all who needed help, but the length of their stay depended on the gravity of their condition.

---

[47] ACB, Hospital de Santa Margarida, Llibres de comptes, 1387–1389, f. 136v.
[48] ACB, Hospital de Santa Margarida, Llibres de comptes, 1379–1380, f. 18v.
[49] ACB, Hospital de Santa Margarida, Llibres de comptes, 1393–1395, f. 56v.
[50] ACB, Hospital de Santa Margarida, Llibres de comptes, 1379–1380, f. 141v, f. 143r–v.
[51] ACB, Hospital de Santa Margarida, Llibres de comptes, 1379–1380, f. 132r.

Conclusions

To sum up some of the most important aspects found in these account books, such as isolation, the relationship between managers and patients or the funding of the hospital, we can analyse the case study of a patient called Jordi. Like Vicens, the slave, he was troublesome and always brought conflict. Compared with other patients, he spent a fair amount of time in the hospital until his death. Although his behaviour (drinking, gambling and even fighting) was as difficult as Vicens's, the most serious problem was his boastfulness.[52]

On the day of Saint Margaret, when parishioners and other citizens went to the hospital church, he talked with some women, bragging about the good life he had at the *leprosarium*.[53] He said that he could come and go as he liked, to the seaside or the vineyards, and that he did not even have to beg for money due to the good funding of the hospital. The manager, outraged, described briefly in the account book the other bad habits of Jordi, such as fighting with the workers or not assisting the other patients with cooking duties.

Jordi was punished, put in chains, and his weekly pay was removed. He responded by protesting, throwing his food and making noise. When new food and his pay were reinstated, he rejected them and stated that he already took some spinach from the orchard. To top the information about this little conflict, we are shown the personality and the temper of one of the patients, and his daily routine on that place.

Undoubtedly, from all the trouble Jordi caused over the years, this was the most serious for the manager. It highlights the dynamics between the managers and the patients, as well as the difference in managerial rules and patient behaviour. Jordi was not supposed to wander around, even though he was expected to beg money for the hospital. This shows that the rules were bent on a regular basis, sometimes even with the knowledge of the manager, that showed a certain tolerance within limits. Jordi was supposed to help at the house and, in fact, there is evidence that he did help, for example, at the orchard. What probably angered the manager the most was Jordi's statement that the hospital had good money. That claim directly endangered the donations and alms, which could not be permitted. It was obvious that a relaxed attitude was allowed, and probably existed with the consent and knowing of the whole city, given that a leper wandering around the city and visiting taverns would attract attention. The fact that Jordi talked with the parishioners exposes a contact with the citizens that until now was deemed

---

[52] ACB, Hospital de Santa Margarida, Llibres de comptes, 1381–1382, f. 51r–51v.
[53] ACB, Hospital de Santa Margarida, Llibres de comptes, 1379–1380, f. 137r–139v.

impossible due to the supposed seclusion of these patients. The limits, though, were the money and survival of the place itself.

The little community of the Hospital of Santa Margarida lived and died no differently than the other hospitals of the city. From day to day, their work tried to improve the lives of those who had nowhere else to go. These account books reveal us how the *leprosarium* was not a place where people were forced to go or to let themselves die. Inside those walls, even the troublesome ones found their share of compassion. When Jordi, the most troublesome of them, died, they had a wake and banquet in his memory, as it was tradition. The same was done for Pau Alemany (German), with additional comments of the manager stating that he was a very good patient and that the wake was held in his loving memory.[54] In the end, all were treated equally.

Bibliography

Albareda, A. 1931. *Història de Montserrat*. Montserrat: Publicacions de l'Abadia de Montserrat.

Brenner, E. 2010. Recent perspectives on leprosy in medieval Western Europe. *History Compass* 8(5): 388–406.

Brodman, J. 1998. Shelter and segregation: lepers and medieval Catalonia, in D. J. Kagay, T. M. Vann (eds), *On the Social Origins of Medieval Institutions: Essays in Honor of Joseph F. O'Callaghan*: 34–45. Leiden: The Netherlands: Brill.

Castellano, A. 1994. L'església de Sant Llàtzer i l'hospital de leprosos de Barcelona a través de la documentació històrica, in *Lambard: Estudis d'art medieval*, no. 6: 41–50. Barcelona: Institut Estudis Catalans.

Conejo, A. 2003. Assistència i hospitalitat a l'Edat Mitjana: L'arquitectura dels hospitals catalans: del gòtic al primer renaixement. Unpublished PhD thesis, Universitat de Barcelona.

Danon, J. 1978. *Visió històrica de l'Hospital General de la Santa Creu de Barcelona*, Barcelona: Rafael Dalmau.

Demaitre, L. 2007. *Leprosy in Premodern Medicine*. Baltimore: Johns Hopkins University Press.

Guilleré, C. 1980. Assistance et charité à Gérone au début du XIVème siècle, in Riu, Manuel (ed.), *La pobreza y la asistencia a los pobres en la Cataluña medieval*, 1: 191–204. Barcelona: CSIC.

Lázaro, R. 1994. La lepra en el Camino Francés a su paso por la Rioja. *IV Semana de Estudios Medievales*, Nájera: 323–340.

---

[54] ACB, Hospital de Santa Margarida, Llibres de comptes, 1389–1391, f. 48r.

Lindgren, U. 1980. *Bedürftigkeit, Armut, Not: Studien zur spätmittelalterlichen Sozialgeschichte Barcelonas*. Münster Westfalen: Aschendorff.
López, A. and Beltran de Heredia, J. 1994. Resultats de l'excavació arqueològica a l'església i a l'hospital de Sant Llàtzer, in *Lambard, Estudis d'art medieval*, no. 6: 51–71. Barcelona: Institut Estudis Catalans.
Pérez Santamaría, A. 1980. El hospital de San Lázaro o Casa dels Malalts o Masells, in Manuel Riu (ed.) *La pobreza y la asistencia a los pobres en la Cataluña medieval*, 1: 75–116. Barcelona: CSIC.
Rawcliffe, C. 2006. *Leprosy in Medieval England*. Woodbridge: Boydell Press.
Triay Olives, V. 2007–2009. *Archaeological Report*. Servei d'Arqueologia de Barcelona, viewed 29 July 2017, <http://cartaarqueologica.bcn.cat/939>.
Villagrasa, E. R. 2015. Hospitales y asistencia en Monzón y el Cinca Medio (siglos XIII–XVI), *Cuadernos CEHIMO*, no. 41: 181–237.

Languages of Experience:
Translating Medicine in MS Laud Misc 237

Lucy Barnhouse

Even as the study of medieval medicine expands, recapturing medieval medical practice as a serious subject in its own right can prove surprisingly difficult.[1] Too often, the theory and practice of medieval medicine have been treated as separate subjects.[2] Though medieval hospitals have been cleared of charges that they were 'not real hospitals', or even 'decrepit and ominous', further studies on therapeutic practice within them remain a desideratum.[3] The absence of doctors, the most readily identifiable practitioners of medieval medicine, from hospitals, the most readily identifiable spaces dedicated to the provision of care, has been treated either as a deficiency or as an enigma.[4] Surveying French and German evidence

---

[1] Park (1991: 26) has justly observed that historians of medieval medicine have often been 'anxious to isolate modern medicine from its benighted past'. Rubin (1991: 14–15) discusses medieval hospitals as multipurpose institutions in which, 'maddeningly', many activities took place that do not fit a modern (Western, clinical, I would add) definition of therapeutic care. Cf. Osborn (2008: 145) for the often-neglected observation that, at the close of the 20th century, over 80 percent of the global population depended on traditional medicine as their primary source of health care. In a similar vein, Riddle (2007: 3–18) has called for the use of comparative anthropology in attempting to assess the accuracy and methods of medieval medicine.

[2] Siriasi (1990), while acknowledging the importance of the social aspects of hospital treatment, views secular and religious ideas of treatment as always separate. Where the implementation of theory has been considered, it has usually been treated as the purview of university-trained physicians. Ballester (1994) outlines developments in late medieval medicine very much as a history of doctors, beginning with the intellectual renaissance (labelled) of the mid-12th century and focusing on the relationship of Aristotelian natural philosophy to academic medicine, and how medicine was practised and conceptualised by these educated practitioners throughout Europe.

[3] The descriptions are taken, respectively, from Imbert (1947: 36) and Allen (2000: 35). Talbot (1955: 169) claims that in the Middle Ages, 'medical science had become stereotyped and fixed', relying on 'threadbare theories and ideas'. Von Steynitz (1970: 18–22) describes medieval hospitals as hampered by a complete lack of hygiene, clean air and water.

[4] Miller (1999: 3–11, 49–50) claims not only that medieval European hospitals were entirely dissociated from the medical profession, but that they were unconcerned with patient

on the structures of care in the medieval hospital, Kay Peter Jankrift concluded that hospital staff simply did not see the service of doctors as essential to their daily functions in the care of the sick-poor.[5] Numerous studies have called for an expanded definition of medieval medicine that would include the management of hospital atmosphere, dietetics and the participation of patients and staff in the liturgy and sacraments of the church.[6]

The eight medical texts collected as a miscellany in the 14th century, and now part of Bodleian MS Laud Misc 237, offer insight into how medicine was understood and practiced in the later Middle Ages. I shall argue that they were used in a hospital community, by both clerical and lay staff. The texts comprising the miscellany—not all previously identified, and not hitherto studied as a group—are classics of medieval university medicine. All in Latin, they include translations of classical and Arabic texts, and works written as part of the western European revival of theoretical medicine in the 12th and 13th centuries. Such texts and their transmission have usually been studied as a field unto themselves: that of learned medicine and its spread among the universities and university-trained doctors of the high and later Middle Ages.[7] But the medical texts in Laud Misc 237 do not appear to have been used by—or even designed for—medical students, professors or university-trained physicians.

---

comfort and health. He contrasts this with Byzantine hospitals, which served as 'nodal points of the medical profession' from the 6th to 13th centuries. See also Von Steynitz (1970: 22–32). McVaugh (2002: 230–245) argues that the increasing presence of doctors in hospitals in the 14th century was rather an indicator of the prestige of the former than changing policies of the latter. McVaugh also finds no evidence for a professional esprit de corps among doctors to accompany the growing number of medical practitioners and the increasing circulation of medical knowledge, both textually and orally.

[5] Jankrift (2007). Jankrift concludes that the absence of doctors from medieval hospital staff was not necessarily a consequence of a dearth of medical professionals. Even in the vicinity of the famous medical school of Montpellier, for example, hospitals showed no noticeable increase in 'medicalization' over their peers elsewhere. In 14th-century Mainz, a physician identified as Magister Otto favored a hospital community in his will, an act consistent with an ongoing relationship; HStAD A2 168/83. The extant documents created by the hospital, however, do not record fees paid to Otto. The term 'sick-poor', nicely approximating the connotations of the Latin *pauperes*, is taken from Sweetinburgh (2004: 12-16 et passim).

[6] See Horden (2007) for an overview. Bonfield (2013: passim), discusses medieval hospitals as environments devoted to holistic healing, and notes that their practices of supplying appropriate food for the sick corresponded to medieval medical theory.

[7] For examples of this rich historiography, see Bos, McVaugh and Shatzmiller (2014: esp. v–viii), Demaitre (2003: 765–788), Jacquart (2004: 399–407) and O'Boyle (2000).

My hypothesis that the collection was used in a hospital rests on the fact that its marginalia contain original medical recipes, prayers to be used as prophylactic and curative medicine, and copious notes on ailments common among the poor and aged, those most often in need of the care provided by medieval hospitals. Users' notes show translation between Latin and the vernacular, between theory and practice, and even, arguably, between practitioners and patients, either of whom might have been only semi-Latinate, if at all. The medical texts of Laud Misc 237 show the languages of theory and experience—and Latin and the vernacular— used in complementary ways, rather than hierarchically. This examination of their use expands on the valuable work done on vernacular medicine in recent years.[8]

Before delving into the contents of the medical miscellany, it is worth turning briefly to the subject of its provenance. Originally created as two miscellanies of four texts each, they were in use by a single community by sometime in the late 14th century. The codex containing the medical texts was in the library of the Cistercian monastery of Eberbach by the 17th century, when Archbishop William Laud arranged its purchase.[9] The monastery's 15th-century library catalogue is not detailed enough to make clear whether or not the codex already existed at that date, or whether the medical miscellanies were then at Eberbach.[10] The medical texts may have been used in the monastery, which managed a hospital, or transferred there from a smaller community under its supervision. Taken together, the marginalia of the medical texts of Laud Misc 237 indicate that they were used in a bilingual community where medicine was studied, taught and administered. By the 14th century, both collections were together (if not yet bound together)

---

[8] On vernacularisation and medical texts, see Voigts (1982). Studies in vernacular medicine have often focused on their uses in domestic, rather than hospital medicine, and on vernacular translations, rather than uses of Latin texts in multilingual environments. See, for example, the work of Theresa Tyers; Lie (2008). This collection, notably, focuses primarily on linguistic questions. Study of the transmission of the Trotula texts has proved illuminating; see, for example, Green (1997); in a similar vein, see Cifuentes (1999). Bennett (2016) is a welcome recent addition to the scholarship on hospital medicine; similar work for Western hospitals is unknown to me.

[9] Coxe and Hunt (1973: 12–14).

[10] Hessisches Hauptstaatsarchiv Wiesbaden Abt. 22 Nr. 436. Rouse and Rouse (1991: 487–494) describe the use of incipits and explicits to enable precise identification; this is, alas, not practised in Eberbach's Oculus Memoriae. Eberbach had all its volumes close at hand. They did not need aids in locating and identifying texts beyond 'A volume of canon law'. These terse identifications, and lack of arrangement by subject, suggest that the Oculus may have been arranged in accordance with the shelving of Eberbach's library *c.* 1500. The number of texts they had would be well explained by service as a lending library, although this remains in the realm of speculation.

and in use in Germany; the hands and orthography found in the marginalia are suggestive of a location in the central Rhineland.

The marginal and interlinear notations on the medical texts of Laud Misc 237 are numerous. Blank folia are covered with detailed original recipes and popular prayers; the diverse marginalia include rubrication to make cures for popular ailments easier to find, and notes on alternative treatments or ingredients. Some of these marginalia are in Latin, and some in German. Moreover, they include several glossaries translating common medical vocabulary from one language to the other. These varied and copious marginalia indicate that some of the manuscript's users were creative as well as knowledgeable practitioners of academic medicine, whether or not they themselves had ever had formal training. All of these characteristics would be consistent with hospital use. Mingled practice of religion and medicine, typical in hospitals, is also implied by a marginal note on the treatise of Hunayn Ibn Ishaq, proclaiming medicine to be a heavenly science, the secrets of which are revealed by the Almighty; more distinctively, if more obscurely, the gloss describes medicine as 'not repudiating the arm of a virgin', presumably from practising it.[11] I have been unable to find any source from which this might have been copied, suggesting that it was intended for the community's nervous novices.

The question of who these novices were may be illuminated by the fact that Laud Misc 237 also contains a vernacular version of the Rule of St Benedict, created for a German-speaking women's house. It is not a direct translation of the Rule, but rather an adaptation designed for a specific community.[12] Significantly, while several sections are omitted from this version of the rule, Chapter 53, on the reception of guests, is here translated as dealing with the treatment of the sick-poor, 'den elenden luden'.[13] Chapter 4, on good works, is rubricated in red and marked with a marginal note 'von den guden werken'.[14] Included in full are the chapters concerning the giving of alms, the services of cooking and laundry—

---

[11] MS Laud Misc 237, fol. 203r. On religious practice as part of therapeutic care, see, for example, Gilchrist (1992: 101); Horden (2001: 135–153); Rubin (1987: 176–182).

[12] MS Laud Misc 237, fol. 1r–fol. 16v. It is a sophisticated work; the prologue on fol. 1r addresses the women as 'Vornemer lieber suster' and opposes them rhetorically to the 'bose dirnen' of the parable of the wise and foolish maidens. Several such adaptations for women's communities exist; see Crean (1993) and Selmer (1933: i–vii).

[13] MS Laud Misc 237, fol. 13v. This section of the rule is twice labelled 'von den elenden luden', but corresponds to a single chapter in the Latin text.

[14] MS Laud Misc 237, fol. 3r. Although the chapter is not translated in its entirety, the section on the works of mercy is kept: 'der armen laben den nakethen cleiden den sichen wisen den doden begraben zu allen noten helffin den swermutdigen trusten'.

crucial to a hospital—and the treatment of sick sisters.¹⁵ To identify the women following that Rule with the community concocting the recipes of the medical miscellany must remain a speculative endeavour; the proximity of the texts, combined with the customisation of each, is suggestive. Moreover, a page from a hospital account book, used as a binding for another Eberbach manuscript in the Laudian collection, makes clear that the monastery's dependencies included at least one women's community responsible for the management of a hospital.¹⁶

Both glosses on the medical texts of Laud Misc 237, and directions in original recipes, indicate that at least some users of the miscellany were expected to be involved in making medicines without a theoretical background in the subject.¹⁷ Therapeutic practices in medieval hospitals were consistent with medical theory, but sophisticated theory and arcane knowledge do not appear to have been the most valued attributes of Laud Misc 237. Rather, cures for joint ailments, headaches and fevers are most frequently highlighted, suggesting that common ailments were the community's chief concern. The miscellany's users also added original recipes. Characteristic is one for oximel, a cough medicine.¹⁸ The recipe, written on the blank verso of the miscellany's first folio, directs the would-be maker of medicines to take cowslips and honey, and boil them in hot water 'the same way you would salt-fish . . . until the decoction is perfect'. The recipe author seems to have thought it wise to clarify this instruction, as being perfect is then described as 'hanging in a thread from the bowl of a small spoon'.¹⁹ Such recipes, appearing alongside sophisticated academic texts, can reveal much about how medieval medicine was practiced and understood.

---

¹⁵ MS Laud 237, fol. 8r, corresponding to Chapters 35 and 36. Also notable is that Chapter 50 is retained, rubricated as 'die suster die uz arbeident', indicating the assumption that some of the sisters will be working outside the cloister; see fol. 11v.

¹⁶ MS Laud Misc 102, fol. 1. The codex itself was produced in the 12th century, but the relevant folio, recording events from the early 14th century, was obviously put in much later. Archbishop Laud's acquisition of the volume in the first third of the 17th century provides only a distant *terminus ante quem*.

¹⁷ On medical theory and hospital environments, see Horden (2001: 147–153) and Rawcliffe (1998).

¹⁸ Getz (2010: 3–4, 24, 35). Oximel was well known enough to feature in satires of medicine; Voigts (2010: 119).

¹⁹ MS Laud Misc 237, fol. 172v: 'Et colatine adde [these words also traced over in later pen] mell(e). lb iiii (4). et b(e)n(e) ibi s(upe)r tr(i)a fin(um) que ponatur super ignem simil(iter) . . . post ea fac bullire tantum ut pisces marini ut fuisset cocti. Post ea excola. et item illam colatam pone s(upe)r ignem [et] | fac decoq(ui)re usque ad perfec(ta)m decoctionem Id est ut de ore cocleari p(ar)vo diffellet filando.'

The medical texts of Laud Misc 237, while they appear to have been used by a single community, were not originally created as a single miscellany. Judging by the wear to the parchment, as well as the page layouts and the hands of the manuscript, I believe the texts fall into two groups. The first, containing three short treatises and a fragmentary prologue, I believe to have been created by an educated member of the hospital where it was used. The first folio of this quire is headed 'Liber de Medicine'. This has led some cataloguers to the conclusion that it contains a single text, but the designation of the 'book of medicine' is that of the copyist.[20] The second collection of texts has a similar generic heading, 'Liber de Medicinis'. Its initial folio clearly served as a cover, being not only worn and stained, but torn and stitched back together.[21] My hypothesis is that both collections, before being bound into the codex of MS Laud 237, were used within the same hospital. The first treatise of the first 'book of medicines' is Gilles de Corbeil's *De Urinis*. This verse text was influential in university circles—and, as this miscellany shows, beyond them.[22] Interlinear notations on the texts clarify their content, apparently serving as memoranda. Amplified descriptions of likely combinations of symptoms are also included among the text's marginalia.[23] Signs of unusually heavy wear appear on Gilles's commentary on the six non-naturals: some of it has been traced over, while the rest is rubbed as if readers' fingers, as well as their eyes, had followed the text.[24]

The second treatise is the *De dosibus medicinarum* of Walter Agilon, who taught at Montpellier in the first half of the 13th century.[25] Notably, it includes a prologue on the nature of medicine, distinct from Agilon's own incipit.[26] This original prologue is the only text in Laud Misc 237 which I have been unable to confidently identify; it may have been an original flourish by the copyist, or adapted from a table of contents to a separate work, which the copyist had but did not use. Agilon's sophisticated and popular medical text is annotated to facilitate

---

[20] Coxe and Hunt (1973: 859).
[21] MS Laud Misc 237, fol. 203r.
[22] Ausécache (1998); O'Boyle (1998: 275); Prioreschi (2003: 258–260).
[23] MS Laud Misc 237, fol. 173r–185v.
[24] MS Laud Misc 237, fol. 173r. On the six non-naturals, see Ballester (2002: 35–42); on the implementation of this theory, Horden (2007: 133–147) is crucial. Park (1991: 37–38) discusses how hospital account books demonstrate practical concern with heating, food and drink, and cleanliness. See also Henderson (2006: 34–67).
[25] O'Boyle (1998: 113–114). This treatise was a popular supplement to the *Ars Medicinae* in medical curricula of the 13th and 14th centuries.
[26] MS Laud Misc 237, fol. 186r. For work on prologues, see Jerman (2011); Black (2012: 153–186) discusses how such prologues could function as independent carriers and interpreters of medical knowledge.

its practical use. Notes such as 'this is to be given weekly to young persons' can, I believe, be read as a sort of dialogue between author and annotator, translating prescription into practice.[27] Here, too, the manuscript's users have included original content. A section on 'simples' contains detailed descriptions of plants and their uses. Such descriptions are consistent with mixed use by experts and non-experts; the manuscript may have served as a reference guide in harvesting plants, as well as in compounding medicines.[28] Among the numerous recipes in the margins are notes on the efficacy of ferns as a purgative, and against melancholy; on spurge as an ingredient in recipes to treat sciatica and skin irritations; and on the uses of a tree root against head colds.[29] These details suggest ailments likely to be exacerbated by age and poverty, and thus infirmities common among those most likely to have recourse to a hospital.[30] That such were the chief concerns of the manuscript's users is confirmed by the marginalia on the third treatise.

---

[27] MS Laud Misc 237, fol. 187r: 'tempore he(bdomad)is in iuvenili etate'.

[28] MS Laud Misc 237, fol. 187v, goes as far as directing what stage of growth roots should be allowed to reach before picking for maximum effectiveness, and includes a scrupulously detailed description of the types of mushrooms that should be taken for medicinal use. Such practices would be consistent with use in a hospital; on hospitals and their gardens, see Meyvaert (1986: 23–31) and Harvey (1992); Rausch (1978: 108–109, 161–168) draws the inference that hospitals normally used plants from their own gardens in the creation of medicines and the provision of care. Diepgen (1911: 55–80) has an index of plants used by Walter Agilon in his *Summa Medicinalis* and a discussion of the ways he most commonly uses them; the commentary of MS Laud Misc 237 appears to be original rather than derivative.

[29] MS Laud Misc 237, fol. 187v–188v.

[30] Agrimi and Crisciani (1998: 170–176) suggest that *infirmitas* was viewed as, in some degree, the natural condition of fallen humanity—or at least a short step away—rather than a category defined against a norm of robust health. Talbot (1955: 172–173) briefly discusses the medieval conceptualisation of sickness as extending to embrace the impoverished and the aged; Sweetinburgh (2004: 1–18, esp. 12–16) observes that the medieval *pauperes* were a vast and broadly construed group including those affected by all sorts of sickness, weakness and social vulnerability. It was through service to this group that medieval hospitals drew their legal as well as their social identity. Sonderegger (2013: 210–212, 214) notes that, for hospitals, taking on corrodians was often a financial loss, and was one of several means by which individuals could claim permanent shelter and care from hospitals, sometimes in exchange for a gift made in advance. Sonderegger is unusual in avoiding an anachronistic distinction between those who entered hospitals in their old age and the other sick-poor. Jankrift (2000: 32–33) points out that old age itself might be more often measured in infirmity than in years. This concept is borne out by a moralising story that appears as part of MS Laud Misc 237 fol. 95v–96r: it treats of an old monk who resists being cared for when sick, behaviour that is treated as sinful and abnormal.

Ricardus Anglicus's *De Repressivis*, a section of his longer *Micrologus*, is glossed with brief explanatory notes.[31] These notes describe what the preparations in the text are good for, and sometimes how they function, as in the case of a recipe which promises to relieve arthritis 'gently and without harm'. Two different hands have used the text in similar ways, adding recipes to the margins. These recipes use plants widely available in the central Rhineland, and include instructions detailed enough to be used by an inexperienced maker of medicines, such as the amount that a liquid should be expected to reduce.[32] The fourth text in the hospital-created collection, and the most heavily glossed, is Gerard of Cremona's *De Clisteribus syringis et pessariis*.[33] I am tempted to characterise it as 'adapted', as the marginalia by turns clarify, amplify and limit the uses suggested in the main text. The marginalia also serve the purpose of making the main text intelligible to users unfamiliar with the medical learning it takes for granted. Notes on Gerard's recipes indicate that one 'gives sleep', and another may be used 'against dry coughs'; or identify a group of treatments as 'the ones we give in pastes [*in pestium*]'.[34]

The next four medical texts, which I consider as a set, show similar signs of practical use, in both their marginalia and their condition. Wide margins are left throughout; pencil sketches in the margin of the first folio suggest that a decorative border may have been envisioned, but in any event, the margin has been filled up with recipe notes. The remaining margins are similarly treated, with many of them completely filled with dense script, in 14th- and 15th-century hands, in both German and Latin. The four texts composing the book are tabbed for easy access, supporting the indication of the marginalia that they were used, as well as designed, as a compendium. The four texts are the *Introductio ad artem parvam* of Johannitius (Hunayn Ibn Ishaq), the *Aphorisms* of Hippocrates, the *Prognostications* of Hippocrates, and Theophilus's *De Urinis*, all of which belonged to the core texts of the *Ars Medicinae* as taught in medical schools of the later Middle Ages.[35] The use of this manuscript, however, appears to have been primarily non-elite.

---

[31] On MSS of the 'De Repressivis', see Thorndike and Kibre (1963: 83); on the identification of Ricardus Anglicus, see O'Boyle (1998: 108).

[32] MS Laud Misc 237, fol. 172r contains instructions on reduction in several original recipes: 'iteris colet(ur) et omnia ista fia(nt) ex quartis ii. aq(ua) et dimidia. ita ut remaneat dua quarta de iste potione'; 'coquntur in tuna sext(er)ia aqua et dimidia | ita ut fra decoctum remanea una sexteria.' See Totelin (2009: 225–258) on the argument that such instructions indicate use by mixed audiences.

[33] Thorndike and Kibre (1963: 228). Minuzzi (2016) speaks of Gerard's text as a key link in medical popularisation.

[34] MS Laud Misc 237, fol. 196v.

[35] See O'Boyle (1998: 271); Löfstedt (2003: 119–21); Siraisi (1981: 98–99, 103–107). For evidence on the use of these texts in universities from Cambridge to Montpellier to Bologna, see

There is less distinction in this collection than in the first in how the different texts are used; marginalia are copied continuously across texts in several places, and are more often independent from the text than those in the first set of treatises. Particularly interesting are the Latin-German glossaries for body parts and the names of plants and herbs. The first of these, on parts of the body, has all entries in the same hand, but not all possible synonyms are grouped together.[36] This appears to indicate a scribe working from multiple sources, adding the different Latin words for, e.g., chest and stomach from different texts or labelled images. The use of *idem* and simplifying tendencies in translation (sometimes with loss of accuracy from Latin to German) suggest that the primary text user is imagined to be Latinate, interacting with non-Latinate persons, whether patients, students, staff or some combination of these.[37] Interaction between the text's users and others is suggested by a marginal note that illnesses might be caused or exacerbated by excessive dampness in the building materials of a dwelling.

Marginalia concerning illnesses caused by an excess of moisture or dryness, cold or heat, often take on a didactic tone. What they attempt to teach are not detailed medical procedures, however, but rather principles of correcting 'sicknesses of cold' with a warm diet, or dry sicknesses (such as fever) with baths.[38] The marginalia's definitions of illness and health may seem, at first glance, to be purely theoretical, but the signs discussed in them could well have been used to determine the standards of admittance for a hospital. The theory that treatment of the sick-poor was a priority for the manuscript's users is supported by the numerous marginal notes on 'paralysis' and various joint ailments; archaeological studies have shown that osteoarthritis was a common affliction among those buried

---

Bullough (2004).

[36] MS Laud Misc 237, fol. 219v–220r. Some of the words, but not all, are grouped in a rough sequence. A second term for nostrils is added as if as an afterthought: De nomibus corporum. Anima vel afla sele . Homos(us) homunculus hominico vel hominuncolus mennelin . Calvaria gekel . oculus auge . ocellus augelin . pupilla augappel . mala wange . maxilla kinebacke vel mandibula. austiria orsmer . auricava orgrube . pinnilla superior pars auris pirula extremitas narium . p(ri)sciores d(icu)n(tu)r antiores dentes palatum slunt sublingum rache . Reniorum inferiorum pars gueturis frumorum superiorum . St(o)ma crop, Volabal index vel solitarius Muffinger . anularis goltfing(er). auricularis orfinger . Corium leder . Sepnui unfleth . aruicia siner. sagine(m) smalz . Sulfur swebil . spina ruckebein . Coxa dich . Sura wade . Tybia knischibe | Cancerium bzant . omai(us) vel vent(er) b(a)uch . luse(us) vel st(oma)co schilender . anas naseloser.'

[37] MS Laud Misc 237, fol. 206v. The most notable pattern is 'Cervix–halsader; fibra–idem; vena–idem; ateria–idem'.

[38] MS Laud Misc 237, fol. 204v, fol. 224r–v.

in hospital cemeteries.³⁹ A religious environment like that of a hospital is also indicated by the fact that the most handled folio in the *Aphorisms* of Hippocrates has its entire margin filled with close-written script, invoking the protection of God in what could be used as a prophylactic or a healing prayer. It includes a 4th-century hexameter catalogue of the names of Christ, 'De Cognomentis Salvatoris', and also a section praying that the person for whom the prayer is said may not suffer harm from the clouds, wind, ether, sun, moon, stars and planets, or dews: a comprehensive catalogue of malign elemental influences!⁴⁰ Following this flamboyant and elaborate prayer, the marginalia return, in contemporary hands, to their usual preoccupations. Original recipes are provided for headaches, fevers, bad breath and eye ailments. Several different hands appear, suggesting the possibility of varying expertise among the annotators.

The *Prognostics* of Hippocrates, succeeding the *Aphorisms,* has most of its margins filled with vocabulary—primarily, but not exclusively, medical. Several pages appear designed to function as a Latin thesaurus, perhaps intended to help a non-Latinate user gain a more sophisticated vocabulary; the same hand responsible for the thesaurus created a Latin/Middle High German dictionary on two subsequent leaves, covering family relationships, parts of the body, healing plants and, intriguingly, buildings: church, library, oratorium and 'the dwellings of the poor' (*magalia, schapstal*). The fact that the community using Laud Misc 237 expected to need words both for buildings typical of religious communities, and for the residences of the poor, vulnerable to disease, is further suggestive of the medical texts' use in a hospital. These places, in other words, were those which the texts' users were expected to describe, among which they were expected to navigate, and to direct others. On the last text in the collection, Theophilus's *De Urinis,* there are brief marginalia summarising Theophilus's conclusions on discolorations of the urine, but the users of the manuscript appear more interested in adding their own recipes for the imbalances he describes.

I argue that the most plausible location for the use of Laud Misc 237's medical texts is a hospital, where staff with varying degrees of theoretical knowledge and practical experience would have ministered to the sick-poor in a religious community.⁴¹ Many of the original recipes assume that their administration will take place as part of a closely observed and controlled regimen. They also

---

[39] Gilchrist (1992: passim; 2005: 202–213); Knüsel, Kemp and Budd (1995).
[40] On the prayer and its uses, see Smith (1976: 195–196); Weyman (1975), 59–61.
[41] Strocchia (2013: 67–92, esp. 77–78) discusses how lay hospital staff would have learned specialised tasks in the course of their labours. She also theorises that women joining hospital staff comparatively late in life would have brought with them years of experience with domestic medicine.

presume the ready availability of bathing facilities. Notes such as 'use parsley and other diuretic herbs' suggest both medical knowledge, and a garden designed for therapeutic purposes, such as was common to medieval hospitals. The marginalia also include directions on when medicine is to be administered, and on cases where preparations should be used immediately after their creation. These all indicate a well-equipped community, usually concerned with common ailments, many of which would be especially common among the poor and aged.

The medical texts of Laud Misc 237 reveal a great deal about the kind of community that used them: a community where recipes were adapted and devised to support holistic regimens; where those knowledgeable in medical theory worked in cooperation with those who used the instruction that a medicine was ready 'when it hangs in a thread from the bowl of the spoon', or advice to 'cook a young chicken and barley with this', as in the marginalia on the treatise of Gerard of Cremona.[42] Latin-German glossaries point to the challenge of translating an academic text into the spoken word, making its healing powers intelligible, as well as manifest. The environment of this medical miscellany was one where theory and practice did not move in separate spheres, but interacted with each other in the work of a variety of practitioners. The marginalia of Laud Misc 237's medical miscellany reveal how medical theory could be implemented through regimens of carefully chosen foods, baths and rest. The community using the miscellany acted to translate theory into practice, Latin into German, providing an environment where medicine, in all its complexities, could be made perfect.

Acknowledgements

I am grateful to Sarah Bull for the opportunity to present an early version of this paper as part of a panel on Languages of the Medical Book at the 2016 meeting of the Society for the History of Authorship, Reading, and Publishing. I am also indebted to Kristin Uscinski for her perceptive and helpful comments on an article draft.

Archival Materials

Hessisches Staatsarchiv Darmstadt A2 168/83
Bodleian Library MS Laud Misc 237
Hessisches Hauptstaatsarchiv Wiesbaden Abt. 22 Nr. 436

---

[42] MS Laud Misc 237, fol. 197v, 'coquere pullum cum ordio'.

Bibliography

Agrimi, J. and Chiara Crisciani, C. 1998. Charity and aid in medieval Christian civilization, in M. D. Grmek (ed.), *Western Medical Thought from Antiquity to the Middle Ages:* 170–196. Cambridge (MA): Harvard University Press.

Allen, P. L. 2000. *The Wages of Sin: Sex and Disease, Past and Present.* Chicago: University of Chicago Press.

García Ballester, L. 1994. Introduction to *Practical Medicine from Salerno to the Black Death:* 1–29. Cambridge: Cambridge University Press.

García Ballester, L. 2002. The origin of the six non-natural things in Galen, in J. Arrizabalaga *et al.* (eds), *Galen and Galenism: Theory and Medical Practice from Antiquity to the European Renaissance*: 35–42. Farnham: Ashgate.

Bennett, D. 2016. *Medicine and Pharmacy in Byzantine Hospitals: A Study of the Extant Formularies.* London: Routledge.

Black, W. 2012. I will add what the Arab once taught: Constantine the African in European medical verse, in A. Van Arsdall and T. Graham (eds), *Herbs and Healers from the Ancient Mediterranean through the Medieval West*: *Essays in Honor of John M. Riddle*: 153–186. Farnham: Ashgate.

Bonfield, C. 2013. Therapeutic regimes for bodily health in medieval English hospitals, in L. Abreu and S. Sheard (eds), *Hospital Life: Theory and Practice from the Medieval to the Modern*, 21–48. Oxford: Peter Lang.

Bos, G., McVaugh, M., and Shatzmiller, J. 2014. *Transmitting a text through three languages: The future history of Galens Peri Anomalou Dyskrasias.* Philadelphia: American Philosophy Society.

Bullough, V. 2004. *Universities, Medicine and Science in the Medieval West.* Farnham: Ashgate.

Cifuentes, L. 1999. Vernacularization as an intellectual and social bridge: The Catalan translations of Teodorico's *Chirurgia* and of Arnau de Vilanova's *Regimen sanitatis*. *Early Science and Medicine: A Journal for the Study of Science, Technology and Medicine in the Pre-Modern Period* 4: 127–148.

Coxe, H. O. and Hunt, R. W. 1973. *Catalogi codicum manuscriptorum Bibliothecae Bodleianae partis secunda codices Latinos et Miscellaneos Laudianos complectens.* Oxford: Bodleian Library.

Demaitre, L. 2003. The art and science of prognostication. *Early University Medicine, Bulletin of the History of Medicine* 77: 765–88.

Diepgen, P. 1911. *Gualteri Agilonis Summa Medicinalis.* Leipzig: Puschmann Stiftung.

Getz, F. M. (ed. and trans.) 2010. *Healing and Society in Medieval England: A Middle English Translation of the Pharmaceutical Writings of Gilberts Anglicus.* Madison: University of Wisconsin Press.

Gilchrist, R. 1992. Christian bodies and souls: The archaeology of life and death in later medieval hospitals, in S. Bassett (ed.), *Death in Towns: Urban Responses to the Dying and the Dead, 100-1600*: 101-118. Leicester: Leicester University Press.

Gilchrist, R. 2005. *Requiem: The Medieval Monastic Cemetery in Britain*. London: Museum of London Archaeology Service.

Green, M. H. 1997. A handlist of the Latin and Vernacular manuscripts of the so-called Trotula texts. Part II: The vernacular texts and Latin re-writings. *Scriptorium* 51: 80-104.

Harvey, J. 1992. Westminster Abbey: The infirmarer's garden. *Garden History* 20: 97-115.

Horden, P. 2001. Religion as medicine: Music in medieval hospitals, in P. Biller and J. Ziegler (eds), *Religion and Medicine in the Middle Ages*: 135-153. Rochester (NY): York Medieval Press.

Horden, P. 2007. A non-natural environment: Medicine without doctors and the medieval European hospital, in B. S. Bowers (ed.), *The Medieval Hospital and Medical Practice*: 133-147. Farnham: Ashgate.

Imbert, J. 1947. *Histoire des hôpitaux français: contribution à létude des rapports de léglise et de l'état dans le domaine de lAssistance Publique: les hôpitaux en droit canonique du décret de Gratien à la sécularisation de ladministration de lHôtel-Dieu de Paris en 1505*. Paris: J. Vrin.

Jacquart, D. 2004. Médicine et philosophie naturelle à Salerne au XIIe siècle, in P. Delogu and P. Peduto (eds), *Salerno nel XII secolo: Istituzioni, società, cultura. Atti del convegno internazionale, Raito di Vietri sul Mare, Auditorium di Villa Guariglia, 16-20 giugno, 1999*: 399-407. Salerno: Incisivo Industrie Graphice.

Jankrift, K. P. 2007. Herren Kranke, arme Siechen. Medizin im spätmittelalterlichen Hospitalwesen, in N. Bulst and K.-H. Spiess (eds), *Sozialgeschihte mittelalterlicher Hospitäler*: 149-167. Ostfildern: Jan Thorbecke Verlag.

Jankrift, K. P. 2000. Vieillir parmi les morts vivants. La léproserie, hospice pour habitants non lépreux?, in B. Tabuteau (ed.), *Lépreux et sociabilité du Moyen Age aux temps modernes*: 31-37. Rouen: Publications de l'Université de Rouen.

Jerman, M. F. L. 2011. A Corpus of Middle English Medical Prologues in the Sloane Collection of the British Library: An Introduction to the Genre in Prose. Unpublished PhD thesis, Universidad de Las Palmas.

Knüsel, C. J., Kemp, R. L., and Budd, P. 1995. Evidence for remedial medical treatment of a severe knee injury from the Fishergate Gilbertine monastery in York. *Journal of Archaeological Science* 22: 369-384.

Lie, O. S. H. Women's medicine in Middle Dutch, in M. Goyens, P. De Leemans, and A. Smets (eds), *Science Translated: Latin and Vernacular Translations of Scientific Treatises in Medieval Europe*: 449-466. Leuven: Leuven University Press.

Löfstedt, B. 2003. Notizen zur Ars Medicinae, *Acta Classica* 46: 119-121.

McVaugh, M. R. 2002. *Medicine Before the Plague: Practitioners and their Patients in the Crown of Aragon, 1285-1345*. Cambridge: Cambridge University Press.

Meyvaert, P. 1986. The medieval monastic garden, in Elisabeth Blair Macdougall (ed.), *Medieval Gardens*: 23-31. Cambridge (MA): Harvard University Press.

Miller, T. S. 1999. *The Birth of the Hospital in the Byzantine Empire*. Baltimore: Johns Hopkins University Press.

Minuzzi, S. 2016. Fifteenth-Century Vernacular Regimen Sanitatis in Verse: Author, Printers, and Readers of Cibaldone. Presentation at the Annual Meeting of the Society for the History of Authorship, Reading, and Publishing, Paris.

O'Boyle, C. 1998. *The Art of Medicine: Medical Teaching at the University of Paris, 1250-1400*. Leiden: Brill.

O'Boyle, C. 2000. Discussions on the nature of medicine at the University of Paris, ca. 1300, in J. Van Engen (ed.), *Learning Institutionalized: Teaching in the Medieval University:* 197-227. Notre Dame (IN): Notre Dame University Press.

Osborn, M. 2008. Anglo-Saxon ethnobotany: Women's reproductive medicine in Leechbook III, in P. Dendle and A. Touwaide (eds), *Health and Healing from the Medieval Garden:* 145-161. Woodbridge: Boydell Press.

Park, K. 1994. Healing the poor: Hospitals and medical assistance in Renaissance Florence, in J. Barry and C. Jones (eds), *Medicine and Charity Before the Welfare State*: 26-45. London: Routledge.

Rausch, U. 1978. *Das Medizinal- und Apothekenwesen der Landgrafschaft Hessen-Darmstadt und des Grossherzogtums Hessen: unter besonderer Berücksichtigung der Provinz Starkenburg*. Darmstadt: Hessische Historische Kommission.

Rawcliffe, C. 1998. Hospital nurses and their work, in I. Britnell (ed.), *Daily Life in the Late Middle Ages*: 43-64. Stroud: Sutton.

Riddle, J. 2007. Research procedures in evaluating medieval medicine, in B. S. Bowers (ed.), *The Medieval Hospital and Medical Practice*: 3-18. Farnham: Ashgate.

Rouse, M. and Rouse, R. 1991. *Authentic Witnesses: Approaches to Medieval Texts and Manuscripts*. Notre Dame (IN): University of Notre Dame Press.

Rubin, M. 1991. Imagining medieval hospitals: Considerations on the cultural meaning of institutional change, in J. Barry and C. Jones (eds), *Medicine and Charity Before the Welfare State*: 14-25. London: Routledge.

Siriasi, N. 1990. *Medieval and Early Renaissance Medicine: An Introduction to Knowledge and Practice*. Chicago: University of Chicago Press.

Siriasi, N. 1981. *Taddeo Alderotti and His Pupils: Two Generations of Italian Medical Learning*. Princeton (NJ): Princeton University Press.

Smith, M. 1976. *Prudentius' Psychomachia: A Reexamination*. Princeton (NJ): Princeton University Press.

Sonderegger, S. 2013. The financing strategy of a major urban hospital in the Late Middle Ages St. Gallen 15th century, in F. Ammannati (ed.), *Assistenza e* solidarietà in Europa Secc. XIII–XVIII = Social Assistance and Solidarity in Europe from the 13th to the 18th Centuries: atti della Quarantaquattresima Settimana di Studi 22–26 aprile 2012: 209–226. Florence: Firenze University Press.

Von Steynitz, J. 1970. *Mittelalterliche Hospitäler der Orden und Städte als Einrichtungen der Sozialen Sicherung.* Berlin: Duncker und Humblot.

Strocchia, S. 2013. Caring for the incurable in Renaissance pox hospitals, in L. Abreu and S. Sheard (eds), *Hospital Life: Theory and Practice from the Medieval to the Modern*, 67–92. Oxford: Peter Lang.

Sweetinburgh, S. 2004. *The Role of the Hospital in Medieval England: Gift-Giving and the Spiritual Economy.* Portland (OR): Four Courts Press.

Talbot, C. H. 1955. *Medicine in Medieval England London*: Oldbourne.

Thorndike, L. and Kibre, P. 1963. *A Catalogue of Incipits of Mediaeval Scientific Writings in Latin.* Cambridge (MA): Mediaeval Academy.

Totelin, L. 2009. Reading, studying, and using the Hippocratic catalogues of recipes. *Studies in Ancient Medicine* 34: 225–258.

Voigts, L. E. 1982. Editing Middle English texts: Needs and issues, in T. H. Levere (ed.), *Editing Texts in the History of Science and Medicine:* 39–67. New York: Garland.

Voigts, L. E. 2010. Herbs and herbal healing satirized in Middle English texts, in A. Van Arsdall and T. Graham (eds), *Herbs and Healers from the Ancient Mediterranean through the Medieval West: Essays in Honor of John M. Riddle*: 217–230. Farnham: Ashgate.

Weyman, C. 1975. *Beiträge zur Geschichte der christlich-lateinischen Poesie.* Hildesheim: Georg Olms Verlag.

Heillög Bein, Brotin Bein:
Manifestations of Disease in Medieval Iceland

Cecilia Collins

In any course on human anatomy and osteology, including palaeopathology, Wolff's Law (1892) remains a foundational concept. According to Wolff's Law, bone is constantly remodelling in response to stressors and forces upon it, whether pathological or activity-induced, so that the bone architecture, shape and robusticity is altered.[1] The interactive process to maintain healthy bone occurs between groups of osteoblast and osteoclast cells. Operating within the basic multicellular unit, osteoclasts resorb diseased or otherwise defunct bone cells, and this activity precedes the work of osteoblasts responsible for the formation of new bone cells.[2] When these cell groups replenish bone cells in a typically healthy individual, this is referred to as normal bone remodelling. The resorption phase lasts approximately for three weeks, while the bone remodelling work of the osteoblasts usually takes three months.[3] When this process is inhibited or suffers from an imbalance due to some disruptive mechanism, the signs remain on the skeleton.[4] Time is therefore also an important component in this system, as the passage of time allows a disease process to enact change on a skeleton. More recent research has offered some necessary clarification to the principles of bone remodelling, especially the ways in which the response differs at various sites and with various stimuli.[5] In younger individuals, i.e., those who are still growing, growth abatement is a common outcome until the stressor is removed or overcome, and for purposes of age estimation, the developmental stages of the dentition and epiphyseal union are the most robust indicators available for ageing juveniles, as their development is less susceptible to such disruptions.[6]

Those unfamiliar with bone architecture and function in living animals and human individuals perhaps tend to think of bone as largely the hard, mineralised component, and thus imagine a skeleton to be only composed of this

---

[1] Pearson and Lieberman (2004: 63); Wolff (1986: 23–24).
[2] Matsuo and Irie (2008: 202).
[3] Matsuo and Irie (2008: 206).
[4] Cf. Aufderheide and Rodriguez-Martin (1998); Ortner (2003).
[5] E.g., Pearson and Lieberman (2004: 65).
[6] Milner and Boldsen (2012: 279).

hard remainder, the stuff of most museum and laboratory encounters. Ancient and medieval peoples, perhaps more than many modern populations, would have understood that the central component of bone, the soft inner marrow, was a nutritious foodstuff. They would have been familiar with the pliability and texture of hand-worked bone to be used as tools or decorative elements. It is this pliability of once-living and dynamic bone upon which palaeopathology has come to rely for registering changes in a skeletonised individual.

Palaeopathology relies on physical descriptors to determine a biological diagnosis. It can be said to be distinct from basic osteological analysis in that it registers more than the basic data of sex, age and measurements, but without such data complementing a pathological diagnosis or description, then certainly the pathological assessment may be of less value. For palaeopathologists, the social context of disease is secondary to the biological phenomenon. This is the legacy of its origins in the field of medicine, where objective evidence is paramount. It is also a function of an understanding that no written records may be available to help contextualise any observed phenomena, or textual witnesses may be scant or otherwise considered unreliable. However, this is not to say that the social context of disease in textual evidence is wilfully ignored; in fact, it is a desired component of any analysis in bioarchaeology that would depict not just the biological phenomena but its contemporary impact.

As a distinct discipline today, palaeopathology has its roots in the work of a few medical practitioners of the 20th century who investigated human remains from archaeological sites with a systematic and clinical approach. In Iceland, Jon Steffensen's work in particular signals the beginning of a crucial shift away from sole reliance on the sagas, settlement records and other texts to relay history, and in particular the history of disease in Iceland.[7] Rather than attempting to peruse the vast body of Icelandic literature available, this paper will attempt to test the congruence of some examples from the literature with pathological conditions which have been identified in some skeletal remains. The hope is to offer a lens through which medieval historians and students of the history of medicine may approach palaeopathology. It is usually ill advised to attempt to diagnose conditions from descriptive texts alone, and by the same turn, not all diseases will leave distinct, pathognomonic marks, if any, on the bones. However, some pathological and/or endemic disease conditions have been reported in medieval and pre-modern Iceland, and have been described in the text in enough detail to allow fairly confident analysis and identification. These conditions will be the focus of this article, while the reader should bear in mind that any attempts to deal with textual authenticity or depictions of the intended audience fall outside of its scope.

---

[7] Zoëga and Gestsdóttir (2011; 203); Gestsdóttir (2012: 548).

According to criteria synthesised by Piers Mitchell, retrospective diagnosis from text works best within a set of optimal parameters for reliability. These include eyewitness testimony, vivid description of the signs and symptoms of disease (including one or more virtually diagnostic symptoms), description of the nature of any lesions and location, little to no evidence for a description which mimics medical views of the period, and finally plausible epidemiological observations in the text.[8] Some of the pitfalls of retrospective diagnosis can include (but are not limited to) a lack of information in the text itself, a researcher's own limited understanding of cultural context, including, for example, the inability to detect that a record which purports to be that of an eyewitness may in fact be a later copy, and finally, an inability to maintain an open mind in thinking outside of a range of modern possible diagnoses or considering that a disease may mutate and change over centuries.[9] In some of the latter examples it is clear that some Icelandic words for certain illnesses were commonly used in the 19th century but fell out of use by the early to mid-20th century. Some terms would certainly have conflated diseases of very different aetiology, and there is no deconstruction of the text possible to attain a retrospective diagnosis in most cases.

Reading in the rich literary tradition from Iceland encompasses the sagas and miracle stories with some reference to local historic annals. Some of the material offers a window into social constructs regarding illness as well as the physical and biological components of the disease experience. Medieval Icelanders believed there were links between emotion and anatomy, especially in a way that can precipitate anatomic changes or differences.[10] Emotional disturbances and strange behaviour, characteristics like timidity or courage, were believed to correlate with the size of one's heart (referring to someone as 'small-hearted' is still commonly used in Icelandic today, and could indicate a sensitive child, for instance). Fear can make one vulnerable to cold, especially when outdoors. In *Eiríks saga rauða*, Sigríður is assisting another woman who has fallen ill. Some have already died of this illness which has swept the farm in Greenland. She experiences coldness and a vision which portends her own death; an illustration of the 'open' body schema of medieval Icelandic beliefs about the body, in which an external element, in this case a draft of cold air, penetrates the body, both conferring illness or disease and acting as an omen of death.[11] This is one of many examples in which not enough information has been transmitted to allow the reader to assume any biological interpretation of these events.

---

[8] Mitchell (2012: 318).
[9] For a complete rundown of potential pitfalls in retrospective diagnosis and how to determine optimal reliability from a source document, see Mitchell (2012: 318).
[10] Kanerva (2014: 228).
[11] Kanerva (2014: 232).

Corporal integrity in archaeology in Iceland

In medieval Icelandic archaeology, the shift parameters towards communal burial can be defined fairly simply. After the settlement period or *landnám* (land-taking), which began in the late 9th century, the entire nation converted to Christianity with a parliamentary motion in the year 999.[12] The archaeology concurs with this dating, as the burials move from a typical pre-Christian Viking mound style in home fields to larger family and community groups being buried in local churchyards.[13] It is believed for this reason that most of the individuals interred in Christian cemeteries are quite representative of the communities once established there. The boundaries of sacred spaces seem largely to have been respected as generally exempt from violence and aggression, for both priests and church properties indicated in 13th-century Iceland.[14]

This immunity of the body did not entirely extend to the grave, as many disarticulated individual remains can attest, though some higher-status graves were excepted, as they seem relatively undisturbed at Skriðuklaustur. Over 260 individuals were recovered from the grounds of the former monastic hospital in east Iceland (1496–1552), and more may remain in the earth. Many disturbed individuals were recovered, including adults and children; preserving the integrity of the deceased's entire corpse was not of paramount importance but it appears to have been at least attempted, when convenient, in a majority of cases. From the burial context, it seems it was considered best to keep individuals in the ground when they were accidentally exposed. However, it does not appear that initial placement was especially important, though an east-west alignment was usually maintained. Thus, articulated limbs were a common find in grave fill or placed alongside other individuals. In one such case, a fully articulated adult individual in Grave 106 was excavated with the vertical upper body and torso of another individual at its foot. Whilst digging a new grave cut, the work most likely exposed the upper portion of this second individual, and so the body was simply tipped upright at the waist.[15]

For medieval Icelanders, bones could be holy relics, and even if these relics were not themselves accessible, powers of transmission were possible. There are examples of *beinavatn*, water in which a saint's relics had been washed, being applied to cure various ailments, including tumours, traumatic injury and even

---

[12] Einarsdóttir (1964: 52).
[13] Vésteinsson (2000: 71).
[14] Jakobsson (2010: 12).
[15] Author's own experience.

vatnormur (see section on *sullaveiki* below).[16] Sigurður Samúelsson's *Sjúkdómar og Dánarmein Íslenskra Fornmanna* (1998) is an excellent source for exploring specific examples from texts, centred around the physician's clinical perspective on descriptions of illness.

Some of the miracle stories indicate an expectation of care by the church that is not just confined to hoping for a miraculous cure. A very early example describes the treatment of 19-year-old Guðmundur Arason, who later became bishop at Hólar. He suffered a broken leg when a ship was stranded during poor weather at sea and was taken to land to be treated by a *læknir*, a term still used in Iceland meaning doctor (here perhaps best understood as a 'healer').[17] The leg did not heal well—*leggja brotin stóðu út úr*—essentially, the leg was set at a bad angle. After some time had passed and Guðmundur had travelled to another part of Iceland, another healer had two men to help him to take bone, the largest *beinflísa* (bone splinters/sequestrum), out of the fracture site, and finally the leg healed well. The period of time from the initial accident to the final healing totalled seven and a half months. About 80 years after his death in 1237, his remains were exhumed with the permission of the bishop at Hólar, and the leg was described as having *hnútarnir mjök stórir sem von var að eftir að brotnaði fótr hans*—very large knots which could be expected after a leg fracture.[18] This text offers some remarkable insights into medical knowledge in a very early period in Iceland. Medical knowledge and healing were evidently practiced in different parts of the country, and healers were trustworthy individuals who are named in the accounts. A broken bone could be set and healed, and healers could even reset badly healed bone and to some degree apply surgical intervention when necessary. Another interesting story of a bone fracture offers less detail, but some tantalising morsels in *Íslendinga saga*: Loftur breaks a foot one summer and finds it to be badly set when healed. Then he allowed it to be broken again and gave his own instructions on how it should be bound—'Lét hann þá brjóta í annat sinn, ok saga sjálfr fyrir hve kinda skyldi.'[19]

Identifying Trauma and Chronic Disease

Traumatic injury is often recognised in the more dramatic examples as above, but traumatic events may produce less pronounced changes, for which the skill of a

---

[16] Skórzewska (2008: 107).
[17] Samúelsson (1998: 220–221) citing *Bysk. II Guðmundar saga Árason* (187, 198). There are a number of interesting elements to the biographies available about Guðmundur biskup, including what could be an early depiction of a migraine headache (Samúelsson 1998: 222).
[18] Samúelsson (1998: 221).
[19] Samúelsson (1998: 130), citing Sturlunga II.b., *Íslendinga saga*, p. 98.

human osteologist is necessary. Injury to and healing of bones in children and adolescents often presents differently than in the adult skeleton and collecting population-level statistics is one of the best means to ascertain how past societies treated their youngest and most vulnerable, and what exposure to particular stressors entailed. In cases of severe illness or trauma, as in the story of Bishop Guðmundur Árason above, bone may die, producing an involcrum of new bone around the dead bone (sequestrum).[20] This is one of the more extreme examples of bone change that may be identified, but even skilled healers could deter the worst possible outcome, as in the case of an example of a femoral fracture in Figure 1; there is obvious asymmetry, but the bone appears to have healed well and without evidence of severe infection. Perhaps a contemporary would also have described these features as *hnútarnir mjök stórir*.

Tuberculosis, treponematoses and leprosy serve as good examples of chronic infection, which have a long duration or recur frequently, and may be identified according to the changes produced, but even these do not always leave evidence on the skeleton. Tuberculosis, for example, is reported to cause skeletal change in only 3 to 7 percent of cases.[21] Many reports on human remains will cite nonspecific

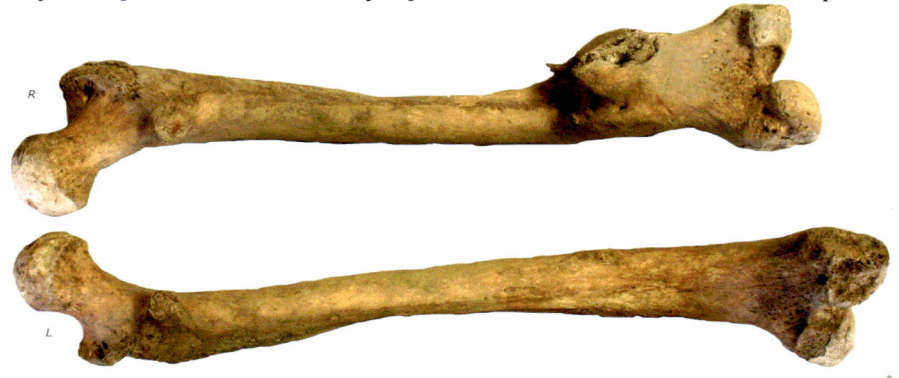

Figure 1: SKR-A-130 Femur
A fractured right femur from an adult male skeleton (SKR-A-130, Skriðuklaustur) has healed but misaligned, leaving it significantly shorter than the left side. Despite this the leg may have been deliberately set and seems to have healed well; there was no evidence of gross infection from this site. Photo by Cecilia Collins.

---

[20] Ortner (2003: 182–185).
[21] Aufderheide and Rodriguez-Martin (1998: 133); Holloway et al. (2011: 403).

infection or inflammation as a diagnosis of bony lesions, as not all pathogens or traumatic events are pathognomonic—i.e., not all leave lesions that can be linked to a specific disease. As the body's first response to pathogens is inflammation, this can appear as pitting of the bone surface (a periosteal reaction), new bone deposition or new woven bone. Thus, even chronic diseases with statutorily accepted diagnostic criteria may be non-specific in early stages of infection and therefore unrecognisable.

Treponemal Disease/*Sárasótt*

Although evidence for treponemal disease in older Icelandic texts is not available, it is important to mention its appearance in the late 15th century in light of the persistent history of controversy surrounding its abrupt emergence in Europe in the Middle Ages. Until the excavation at the monastic site Skriðuklaustur produced evidence of treponemal disease in Icelandic skeletal remains, many believed the disease to have only arrived in Iceland in the 19th century. *Bartskerar*, barber-surgeons, were invited by the bishop Ögmundur Pálsson in 1525 to come to Iceland, and a good tract of farmland was offered as payment for healing the populace from syphilis.[22] However, a belief has persisted among historians that the medieval authors of documents referring to syphilis were confusing the disease with leprosy or scrofula.[23] While there is some possible support for this theory in relation to medieval belief in a venereal transmission of leprosy, this theory has been refuted using evidence from skeletal remains indicating that these conditions could not have been confused.[24]

When identified in human skeletal remains, the changes produced by tertiary syphilis distinctively affect the long bones and the cranium, with the most commonly affected being the tibia and the frontal and parietal bones of the cranium. Other affected bones may include the nasal-palatine region, sternum, clavicle, vertebrae, femur, fibula, humerus, ulna and radius. The gummatous lesions of the skull, also known as *caries sicca*, are very distinctive. These lesions may resemble other conditions such as tumours and tuberculous infection, but differential diagnosis can often solve confusions that may arise. In addition to the changes described above, in cases of congenital syphilis, further distinctive changes to the dentition would be recorded.[25] It is worth noting that syphilitic lesions on a human skeleton represent an advanced stage of chronic disease. The

---

[22] Þórláksson (2003: 124); Ísleifsdóttir (1997: 104).
[23] Ísberg (2005: 162); Þórláksson (2003: 124).
[24] Roberts and Manchester (2007: 213); Crane-Kramer (2002: 117).
[25] Aufderheide and Rodriguez-Martin (1998: 158, 161, 163–164).

condition is known to affect brain function when left untreated and therefore could also impair mental capacity. These circumstances are of course impossible to delineate from human remains alone but bear consideration in the spectrum of disabling and disfiguring disease in social context.

Hydatid Disease/*Sullaveiki*

A study of disease in the past must also carefully consider the human-animal relationship in the past. The greatest consequence of domestication of dogs and sheep and their import to Iceland soon after settlement was the accessory import of a deadly tapeworm. The term *sullur/sullr* refers to a cyst, though its precise aetiology is unclear, and at least from the 19th century onwards the term *sullaveiki* is associated with liquid-filled cysts, sometimes with a fully or partially calcified perimeter. Even in the 19th century, however, many doctors believed these idiosyncratic swellings to be the result of a form of hepatitis unique to colder northern climates, and it was only the work of the Danish doctor Harald Krabbe which undid this misconception; the association with hepatitis was probably due to the parasite's proclivity to cause swelling of the liver.[26] It is certain that a parasitic helminth, *E. granulosus*, became endemic after *landnám* and remained so until the mid-20th century when it was eradicated from Iceland.[27] Described as one of the 'worst and most dangerous diseases in Iceland', hydatid disease, or echinococcosis, appeared with enough frequency in the population to be listed alongside tuberculosis and leprosy as one of the most distressing endemic diseases in Iceland, even at the beginning of the 20th century. Many doctors in the 19th century reported finding cysts during autopsies.[28] Characterised by localised swellings, the condition may impair particular organs and skeletal tissue, and eventuate in death, but may also progress for some years before the victim suffers great discomfort.[29]

The parasite's hosts during its life cycle are dogs and sheep, and humans may be accidentally infected in any area of the body. Transmission is most often a result of fecal-oral contact via the infected waste material of dogs or sheep. The consequences of infection by the worm and its larvae mean that though the liver can normally filter out such infections after accidental ingestion, it may be overwhelmed and is the primary site of infection in 60 percent of cases, followed

---

[26] Krabbe (1864).
[27] Dungal (1946: 12); Richter and Elmarsdóttir (1997: 151).
[28] Jónsson (1900: 89), my translation; Halldórsdóttir (1995: 28, 30).
[29] Arinbjarnar (1989: 402).

by the lungs (30 percent) and other organs/sites in the body.[30] For our purposes, cyst fragments are represented in the archaeological record and can be identified through a process of differential diagnosis. A hydatid cyst of approximately 17–20 cm in diameter, ovoid in shape, was recovered from an elderly female skeleton at Skriðuklaustur, and another example which was perhaps as large as 15 cm in diameter was recovered from an elderly female at Viðey, an island in the greater Reykjavík area.[31] There are a number of miracle stories which very likely refer to infection by this parasite, specifically stories which mention water draining from a puncture site. However, not all references to *sullr* can be definitively tied to this condition, though many are probably linked. A term which appears in the literature, *vatnormur,* meaning literally 'water-worm', can be linked to this condition with some confidence.[32] One may postulate further that *vatnormur* evolved to *sullr* with the caveat that *sullr* entertains a number of diseases which produce swelling. Specific examples are found in Sigurður Samúelsson's book and include the story of Halla Lýtingsdóttir in *Vopnfirðinga saga* (13th century), and the story of a young girl, Árnríðr, in *Jóns saga Hólabyskups ens Helga* XLI, as well as at least three others from *biskupa sögur* (mid-14th century) (though these are somewhat less detailed). Árníðr's story offers an especially useful insight; her father comments that he has recognised such swellings in his animals, and if it were one of his animals, he would puncture the site himself.

Leprosy/*Holdsveiki*: A Conspicuous Absence

Some of the better-known historic examples of leprosy come from the annals concerning the Icelandic bishops and their households, and others such as some of the district sheriffs, beginning in the early 17th century.[33] Known first in *Fornaladarsögum Norðurlanda* as *líkþrá* (*lepra*) and later more commonly as *holdsveiki*, at least four hospitals were established to treat leprosy, all of which were disbanded by 1848 (Skriðuklaustur is not included in this list).[34] Usually, leprosy would be diagnosed in a skeleton by a triad of signs designated as *facies leprosa,* including atrophy of the anterior nasal spine, atrophy and recession of the alveolar processes of the maxillae (the upper jaw), and inflammatory changes which cause the

---

[30] Thaler et al. (2010: 1417–1418).
[31] See Kristjánsdóttir and Collins (2010); Collins (2013); Gestsdóttir (2004: 28).
[32] *Biskupa sögur* III: 445–446; Samúelsson (1998: 34); Skórzewska (2008: 107). Skórzewska is less certain of the origin of the term *vatnormur,* but Samúelsson assesses it confidently as linked to hydatid disease.
[33] Jónssson (1944: 122ff.).
[34] Samúelsson (1998: 28–29).

appearance of receding bone around the maxilla and nasal aperture in conjunction with changes to the hands and feet.[35] However, the skeletal record has yet to yield convincing evidence of this disease in the growing numbers (currently c. 1,300) of skeletons currently curated in Iceland.[36]

The conspicuous absence of leprosy in the skeletal remains from Iceland can be attributed perhaps to the presence of endemic tuberculosis. Although the evidence from later 20th-century medical reports falls outside of the usual scope of a medieval study, some important points regarding the epidemiology and morbidity of disease in a population can cast light on how disease may have exhibited in the past. The medical establishment in the 19th and early 20th centuries recognised that tuberculosis could be reactivated in a person following a latent period, and was believed with treatment (as it was provided in the pre-antibiotic era) to improve of its own accord. Evidence from annual reports in the early 20th century show that after outbreaks of other diseases such as measles, influenza and pertussis, inactive cases of tuberculosis reemerged in the medical reports, and there was a corresponding rise in the number of those being treated for consumption.[37] Palaeopathology has confirmed that skeletal lesions formed during active periods of tuberculosis may heal, sometimes leaving little trace.[38]

Autopsies of 111 cadavers that had been diagnosed with leprosy as a cause of death during the period 1898–1919 found that 46 (41.4 percent) had signs of active or latent tuberculosis.[39] In 1920, the General Surgeon (*Landslæknir*) surveyed 811 patients being treated at the tuberculosis sanatorium in Vífilsstaðir (founded 1910). Of those surveyed, 326 could relate a plausible history of when they first became infected, and 242 of those believed themselves to have contracted tuberculosis in childhood, before the age of 10. In a later report derived from patient interviews (1923), he wrote that he also believed a majority of those infected to have contracted tuberculosis which was transmitted over many generations in their households.[40]

There is also a potential for misdiagnosis of cutaneous facial lesions, particularly in the early stages of leprosy. Differential diagnosis of ulcers or chancre can include syphilitic chancre and *lupus vulgaris* (produced by tuberculosis). In fact, the minutes of the medical council meetings and annual reports from the early 20th century do suggest that such confusion might have been more common

---

[35] Boocock et al. (1995: 265); Ortner (2003: 264; 2008: 202–203). *Facies leprosa* was first described by Möller-Christensen et al. (1952: 336).
[36] Gestsdóttir (2014: 131).
[37] Sigurdsson (1950: 12).
[38] Ortner (2003: 230); Holloway *et al.* (2011).
[39] Bjarnhéðinsson (1919: 148).
[40] As reported in Sigurdsson (1950: 8).

than not, as one doctor even commented that *lupus vulgaris* seems a common tuberculosis manifestation in Denmark but is in his opinion unlikely to be a cause of the disease among Icelanders.[41] Cross-immunity to *M. leprae* in those infected primarily by *M. bovis* or *M. tuberculosis* has been proffered as an answer to the apparent decline of leprosy in Scandinavia, but those primarily infected with *M. leprae* are rather more vulnerable to *M. tuberculosis,* and it is highly likely that these individuals succumbed sooner.[42]

A former head of antiquities in Iceland, *Þjóðminjavörður* Þór Magnússon, in a 1994 newspaper article, described being contacted in 1968 to retrieve remains from an old disused church cemetery at Gufunes, Reykjavík. Sadly, this location was associated with a former leper hospital, and the remains had been scattered across the site during construction work. The photos taken by staff from the National Museum during their rescue effort show that by the time they arrived at the site, all that remained was a large trench of approximately two to three meters' depth and width. These remains numbered approximately 768 individuals and were reinterred without examination at the new church in Gufunes. Only one individual, whose engraved silver coffin nameplate indicated that he had held a number of prominent government positions during his lifetime, including lastly Keeper of the Leper Hospital, remained intact and was then taken to be curated at the National Museum.[43] Interestingly, the skeleton of Páll Jónsson (1737–1819) is only one of a handful of individuals of known age and date in the collection (the remains of some bishops and their family members from Reykholt).

Tuberculosis/*Berklaveiki*

Berklur usually refers to tuberculosis, yet its usage and aetiology prior to the 19th century is more ambiguous in many cases. In its most extreme and most commonly recognised form, tuberculosis predilects the spinal region and causes destruction of the vertebrae, sometimes leading to gibbous deformity, or kyphosis (Figure 2). It is critical to recognise that not all instances of changes to ribs indicate tuberculosis, but when observed can at most be ascribed to a chronic lung infection. In order for tuberculosis to be considered in diagnosis, a certain constellation of changes is necessary (precluding molecular analysis). A classic and most commonly recognised change is kyphosis of the spine, called Pott's disease.[44] Jón Steffensen in the 1939 excavation at Skeljastaðir in Þjórsárdal, southern Iceland, first found tuberculosis

---

[41] Clæssen (1928: 103).
[42] Lynnerup and Boldsen (2012: 467).
[43] Magnússson (1994: 19); Guðmundsdóttir (2004: 14).
[44] Ortner (2003: 230).

of the spine in an Icelandic archaeological context. Since then, the remains from Skeljastaðir have been examined by Hildur Gestsdóttir (2009), who proposed that tuberculosis was endemic in the valley at the time. Changes to individual skeletons indicative of lung infection have been identified at Skeljastaðir, Skriðuklaustur and Hofstaðir.[45]

Literary references to this condition are not so easily disentangled from other conditions, especially pulmonary infections such as pneumonia.[46] The sagas and the remaining parish annals contain references to conditions that insinuate similar symptoms. In cases of possible pneumonia, time to rest seems the greatest factor in recovery, along with a dose of divine intervention in *Jóns saga helga*.[47] Most of the written evidence for tuberculosis in Iceland has been cited from the 17th century and later, the most famous examples being the children and grandchildren of the bishop Brynjólfur Sveinsson (1639–1674) at Skálholt, and of Árni Þórarinsson (1741–1787), bishop at Hólar, who died at 46 years of age of tuberculosis.[48]

Even a recent genetic study of tuberculosis risk among Icelanders has cited the general view that tuberculosis was rare in Iceland until the 19th century.[49] This follows the clinicians' view which has predominated the study of

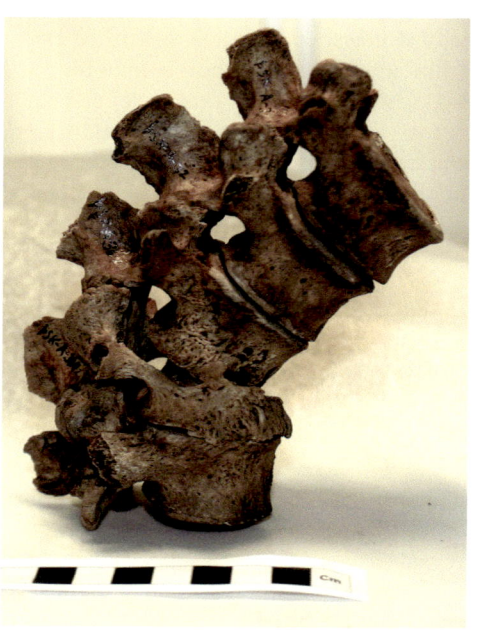

Figure 2: ÞSK-A-32 Lumbar Spine
The lumbar vertebrae from a male skeleton, aged 18-25 years (ÞSK-A-32, Skeljastaðir) are affected by severe tuberculous infection, which has caused Pott's disease of the spine.
Photo by Cecilia Collins.

---

[45] Cf. Collins (2010, 2011, forthcoming); Gestsdóttir (2009); Sundman (2011).
[46] Samúelsson (1998: 65–66) posits *lungnabólga með brjósthimnubólgu*, swelling of the lungs and chest, as a likely description of pneumonia.
[47] Samúelsson (1998: 68), citing Bysk., II. b., *Jóns saga helga*, 122 and Bysk., I.b., *Jarteinabók Þorláks byskup önnur*, 198.
[48] Samúelsson (1998: 35).
[49] Sveinbjörnsson et al. (2016: 483).

historical tuberculosis in Iceland.[50] In his landmark work on depictions of disease in Iceland, Sigurður Samúelsson concurs generally with the view that tuberculosis was not highly prevalent in medieval and pre-modern Iceland. Even though he does give a nod to Steffensen's work, he separates examples of possible tuberculosis from other diseases affecting the lungs. The descriptions of these chronic respiratory diseases, however, could be attributed to tuberculosis and should be considered as a possible aetiology, especially given its highly transmissible nature.[51] The mounting evidence in archaeological remains, from diverse regions of Iceland, also offers rather illustrative proof of its presence in Iceland much earlier than previously thought. Lastly, since Steffensen first identified an extreme case of kyphosis in the remains from Skeljastaðir, advances in palaeopathology have made it possible to identify further pathognomonic lesions which support the case for recognising tuberculosis as an endemic or epidemic disease.

Summary

Finally, a word of caution that the identification of specific infectious disease does not only incorporate a superficially limited suite of diagnostic options. Studying skeletal populations has enriched our understanding of many periods and places in history. A real grasp of health and disease in past lives requires an investment of time and resources to understand the clinical basis of palaeopathology and how the discipline approaches a host of markers of stress, metabolic deficiency and trauma, which even when cited as 'nonspecific' can offer valuable insights. Though at times it seems an imprecise science, palaeopathology can and should shift the lens through which we approach disease and its representations in text. Textual witnesses are now more than ever supplemented by biological and archaeologically contextualised evidence of disease and social practice. Where students of palaeopathology are sometimes limited to reviewing text from relatively recent periods and often without access to the original language, collaborative work with historians can certainly remedy these gaps.[52]

Ongoing palaeopathological analysis of the human remains curated in Iceland thus far finds evidence that the presence of endemic diseases in the population, perhaps introduced even at the settlement of Iceland, may eclipse the presence of other types of infectious disease. Using molecular analysis, the material may present a fascinating opportunity to better understand the interactions

---

[50] Samúelsson (1998: 35); Jónsson (1944: 112).
[51] Samúelsson (1998: 65–66). In some cases *sullaveiki* may have also been the culprit for the sensation of swelling or stinging in the lungs and chest.
[52] Mitchell (2012: 310).

between leprosy and tuberculosis. In the rest of medieval Europe, there was a distinct change from a high leprosy to a high tuberculosis ratio, and there is much direct skeletal evidence for this shift. It would appear that tuberculous infection can confer a degree of immunity to leprous infection.[53] Of course, further recovery of remains in archaeological excavation always holds the possibility to uncover evidence of leprosy or other conditions and any corresponding evidence from textual witnesses is invaluable. Both texts and palaeopathology suggest that medical knowledge was utilised and transmitted, and that retrospective diagnosis is enlightening, perhaps even practical. In the maelstrom of debate regarding the evidence and evidence lacking in the history of disease in Iceland, palaeopathology stands as another witness as current knowledge is expanded and consolidated.

Acknowledgements

The following individuals or institutions provided access to archaeological material: The National Museum of Iceland, Guðný Zoëga at the Cultural Heritage Centre in Skagafjörður, and Hildur Gestsdóttir at the Archaeological Institute of Iceland.

Bibliography

Arinbjarnar, G. 1989. Fjögur Sullatilvik á Fjörðungssjúkrajúsinu á Akureryi 1984–1988. *Læknablaðið* 75: 399–403.

Aufderheide, A. C. and Rodriguez-Martin, C. 1998. *The Cambridge Encyclopedia of Human Paleopathology.* Cambridge University Press.

Bjarnhéðinsson, S. 1919. Frá Laugarnesspítalnum. *Læknablaðið* 5: 145–149.

Boocock, P., Roberts, C., and Manchester, K. 1995. Prevalence of maxillary sinusitis in leprous individuals from a medieval leprosy hospital. *International Journal of Leprosy* 63(3): 265–268.

Callow, C. and Evans, C. 2016. The Mystery of plague in medieval Iceland. *Journal of Medieval History* 42(2): 254–284.

Clæssen, G. 1928. Aðaltundur læknafjelags islands. *Læknablaðið* 14: 101–112.

Collins, C. (forthcoming) 2018. *The Palaeopathology of Maxillary Sinusitis, Otitis Media and Mastoiditis in Medieval Iceland.* Unpublished PhD Thesis. University of Reading.

Collins, C. 2013. The unbidden houseguest: endemic hydatid disease in Iceland. *Archaeological Review from Cambridge* 28(2): 46–61.

---

[53] Lynnerup and Boldsen (2012: 466–467).

Collins, C. 2011. *Osteological Analysis of the Human Remains from Skriðuklaustur, 2010 Excavation Season*. Skýrslur Skriðuklaustursrannsókna [Skriðuklaustur Research Reports].

Collins, C. 2010. *An Osteological Analysis of the Human Remains from Skriðuklaustur, 2009 Excavation Season*. Skýrslur Skriðuklaustursrannsókna xxi. Reykjavík: Skriðuklaustursrannsóknir.

Crane-Kramer, G. M. M. 2002. Was there a medieval diagnostic confusion between leprosy and syphilis? an examination of the skeletal evidence, in C. A. Roberts, M. E. Lewis, and K. Manchester (eds), *The Past and Present of Leprosy: Archaeological, Historical, Palaeopathological and Clinical Approaches*, British Archaeological Reports International Series 1054: 111–119. Oxford: Archaeopress.

Dungal, N. 1946. Echinococcosis in Iceland. *American Journal of Medical Science* 212: 12-17.

Einarsdóttir, Ó. 1964. *Studier í kronologisk metode i tidlig islandsk historieskrivning*. Bibliotheca historica Lundensis, 13. Stockholm: CWK Gleerup.

Gestsdóttir, H. 2004. *The Palaeopathology of Iceland: Preliminary Report 2003: Haffjarðarey, Neðranes &Viðey*. Reykjavík: Fornleifastofnun Íslands.

Gestsdóttir, H. 2009. Sögur af Beinagrindum. *Árbók Hins Íslenzka fornleifafélags 2008-2009*: 123–142.

Gestsdóttir, H. 2012. Historical osteoarchaeology in Iceland. *International Journal of Historical Archaeology* 16(3): 547–558.

Gestsdóttir, H. 2014. Chapter 9, Themes in Icelandic bioarchaeological research: 127–137 in B. O'Donnabhain and M. C. Lozada (eds), *Archaeological Human Remains*. Briefs in Archaeology. New York: Springer.

Guðmundsdóttir, A. L. 2004. *Fornleifaskráning jarðarinnar Gufuness og hjáleigu hennar Knútskots*. Skýrsla nr [Report no.] 115. Reykjavík, Minjasafn Reykjavíkur, Árbæjarsafn.

Halldórsdóttir, E. D. 1995. Skorið á sull og einangrun rotnandi fólks. Sóknin gegn sullaveiki og holdsveiki. *Sagnir* 16: 28–35.

Holloway, K., Henneberg, R., and de Barros Lopes, M. 2011. Evolution of human tuberculosis: a systematic review and meta-analysis of paleopathological evidence. *HOMO-Journal of Comparative Human Biology* 62:402 -458.

Ísberg, J. Ó. 2005. *Líf og lækningar: íslensk heilbrigðissaga*. Reykjavík: Hið íslenska bókmenntafélag.

Ísleifsdóttir, V. A. 1997. *Siðbreytingin á Íslandi 1537-1565*. Reykjavík: Hið íslenska bókmenntafélag.

Jakobsson, S. 2010. Heaven is a place on earth: church and sacred space in thirteenth-century Iceland. *Scandinavian Studies* 82: 1–20.

Jónsson, B. 1900. Dr H. Krabbe og kona hans. *Sunnanfari* 8(12): 89–90.

Jónsson, S. 1944. *Sóttarfar og sjúkdómar á Íslandi 1400-1800*. Reykjavík: Hið íslenska bókmenntafélag.

Kanerva, K. 2014. Disturbances of the mind and body: effects of the living dead in medieval Iceland, in S. Katajala-Peltomaa and S. Niiranen (eds), *Mental (Dis) order in Later Medieval Europe*: 219–42. Leiden: Brill.

Krabbe, H. 1864. *Athugasemdir handa Íslendingum um sullaveikina og varnir móti henni*. Copenhagen: J. H. Schultz.

Kristjánsdóttir, S. 2013. Skriðuklaustur monastery in medieval Iceland: a colony of religiosity and culture, in E. Jamroziak and K. Stöber (eds), *Monasteries on the Borders of Medieval Europe: Conflict and Cultural Interaction*: 149–172. Turnhout: Brepols.

Kristjánsdóttir, S. and Collins, C. 2010. Cases of hydatid disease in medieval Iceland. *International Journal of Osteoarchaeology* 21(4): 479–486.

Lynnerup, N. and Boldsen, J. 2012. Leprosy (Hansen's disease), in A. L. Grauer (ed.), *A Companion to Paleopathology*: 458–471. Chichester: Wiley-Blackwell.

Magnússon, Þ. 1994. Er nú Jón tyndur líka? *Morgunblaðið*, 16 July 1994, p. 19.

Matsuo, K. and Irie, N. 2008. Osteoclast–osteoblast communication. *Archives of Biochemistry and Biophysics* 473(2): 201–209.

Milner, G. R. and Boldsen, J. L. 2012. Estimating age and sex from the skeleton: a paleopathological perspective, in A. L. Grauer (ed.), *A Companion to Paleopathology*: 268–284. Chichester: Wiley-Blackwell.

Mitchell, P. 2012. Integrating historical sources with paleopathology, in A. L. Grauer (ed.), *A Companion to Paleopathology*: 310-323. Chichester: Wiley-Blackwell.

Möller-Christensen, V., Bakke, S. N., Melsom, R. S., and Waaler, E. 1952. Changes in the anterior nasal spine of the alveolar process of the maxillary bone in leprosy. *International Journal of Leprosy* 20: 335–340.

Ortner, D. 2003. *Identification of Pathological Conditions in Human Skeletal Remains*, 2nd ed. Washington, DC: Academic Press.

Ortner, D. 2008. Differential diagnosis of skeletal lesions in infectious disease, in R. Pinhasi and S. Mays (eds), *Advances in Human Palaeopathology*: 191–214. Chichester: John Wiley & Sons.

Pearson, O. M. and Lieberman, D. E. 2004. The ageing of Wolff's "Law": ontogeny and responses to mechanical loading in cortical bone. *Yearbook of Physical Anthropology* 47: 63–99.

Richter, S. H. and Elmarsdóttir, Á. 1997. Intestinal parasites in dogs in Iceland: the past and the present. *Icelandic Agricultural Science* 11: 151–158.

Roberts, C. and Manchester, K. 2007. *The Archaeology of Disease, Third Ed.* Ithaca: Cornell University Press.

Samúelsson, S. 1998. *Sjúkdómar og dánarmein íslenskra fornmanna*. Reykjavík: Háskólaútgáfan.

Sigurðsson, S. 1976. Um berklaveiki á Íslandi. *Læknablaðið* 62: 3–50.

Sigurdsson, S. 1950. *Tuberculosis in Iceland: epidemiological studies.* U.S. Public Health Service Publication No. 21 (Technical Monograph No. 2), Washington, DC.

Skórzewska, J. A. 2008. 'Sveinn Einn Ungr Fell í Sýkúrer': Medieval Icelandic children in vernacular miracle stories, in S. Lewis-Simpson (ed.), *Youth and Age in the Medieval North.* The Northern World, 42: 103–126. Leiden: Brill.

Sundman, E. A. 2011. *Osteological Analysis of the Human Remains— Skriðuklaustur 2011.* Skýrslur Skriðuklaustursrannsókna XXXI. Reykjavík: Skriðuklaustursrannsóknir.

Sveinbjornsson, G., Gudbjartsson, D. F., Halldorsson, B. V., Kristinsson, K. G., Gottfredsson, M., Barrett, J. C. *et al.* 2016. HLA class II sequence variants influence tuberculosis risk in populations of European ancestry. *Nature Genetics* 48(3): 318–322.

Thaler, M., Gabl, M., Lechner, R., Gstöttner, M. and Bach, C. M. 2010. Severe kyphoscoliosis after primary echinococcus granulosus infection of the spine. *European Spine Journal: Official Publication of the European Spine Society, the European Spinal Deformity Society, and the European Section of the Cervical Spine Research Society* 19(9): 1415–1422.

Vésteinsson, O. 2000. *The Christianization of Iceland: priests, power, and social change, 1000–1300.* Oxford: Oxford University Press.

Wolff, J. 1986. *The law of bone remodeling* [translated from the 1892 original, *Das Gesetz der Transformation der Knochen,* by P. Maquet and R. Furlong]. Berlin: Springer Verlag.

Zoëga, G. and Gestsdóttir, H. 2011. Iceland/Ísland, in L. Fibiger and N. Marquez-Grant (eds), *The Routledge Handbook of Archaeological Human Remains and Legislation: An International Guide to Laws and Practice in the Excavation and Treatment of Archaeological Human Remains:* 203–238. London: Routledge.

Þórláksson, H. 2003. *Saga Íslands VI.* Reykjavík: Sögufélag og Hið íslenska bókmenntafélag.

A Case Study of *Plantago* in the Treatment of Infected Wounds in the Middle English Translation of Bernard of Gordon's *Lilium medicinae*

Erin Connelly

In his *Certaine Workes of Chirurgerie*, Thomas Gale (a 16th-century barber-surgeon connected with the provenance[1] of the Middle English translation of the *Lilium medicinae*) related a personal case study of a child with 'sore eyes'. The text states that many medicines and treatments were applied, which only 'brought the eyes to worse'. Eventually, the physicians gave up hope, and the child was 'lefte to the worke of nature'. However, the child's mother found a recipe in 'an olde boke' for Gale to prepare, which restored the child's eyes to 'perfecte helth and sight'.[2] Although Gale's account is several centuries old, it is analogous to a current situation. At present, there is an urgent need for novel routes to drug discovery due to the significant increase in antibiotic-resistant microbes and the lack of new drugs currently in development to treat antibiotic-resistant infections. For instance, the World Health Organization (WHO) stated in September 2016 and 2017 that antimicrobial resistance is 'an increasingly serious threat to global public health that requires action across all government sectors and society' and 'the world is running out of antibiotics'.[3] If no action is taken, it has been estimated that such infections will kill 10 million people a year by 2050.[4] Like Thomas Gale's account of a successful remedy from an 'olde boke', some present-day historians and scientists suggest that answers to the antibiotic crisis may be inspired by medical history in combination with modern technologies. For instance, in 2015, Youyou Tu jointly won the Nobel Prize in Physiology or Medicine for the development of a new therapy (artemisinin) to treat malaria. Significantly, the antimalarial component was extracted from the plant *Artemisia annua* after consulting the instructions found in the 'ancient literature' of traditional herbal medicine.[5] At the same time that she was awarded the Nobel Prize, Harrison *et al.* were investigating

---

[1] Connelly (2017).
[2] All quotes are from Gale (1563); quotes are from fols. 87–88 of the *Antidotarie*.
[3] WHO (2016, 2017).
[4] Review on Antimicrobial Resistance (2014: 5; 2016: 11).
[5] Tu (2011); Nobelprize.org (2015).

a 10th-century Anglo-Saxon remedy for eye infection known as Bald's eyesalve.[6] This remedy from an 'olde boke' was shown to be a potent antibacterial agent with great potential for treating a range of antibiotic-resistant soft tissue pathogens, including the superbug methicillin-resistant *Staphylococcus aureus* (MRSA).[7] It was demonstrated that while the ingredients had little or no antimicrobial activity when acting alone, they were highly effective at killing bacteria when combined as specified in the recipe, which suggests a possible medieval methodology in creating multipartite recipes informed by a long tradition of observation and experimentation. Along those lines, the following discussion will aim to demonstrate the complementary nature of this interdisciplinary research in the selection of potential candidates for laboratory testing. The case study will first provide a brief overview of the significance of the *Lilium medicinae* and its Middle English translation, known as the *Lylye of Medicynes*, and then will present four recipes from the *Lylye* used for treating simple to severe infected wounds and examine what can be learned about their potential candidacy for experimental testing in light of recent scientific studies on the genus *Plantago*.

Bernard of Gordon was a medical doctor and lecturer in Montpellier who completed his most ambitious work, the *Lilium medicinae*, in 1305. Among the list of medical authorities in the *Canterbury Tales General Prologue*, Chaucer cites Bernard alongside Dioscorides, Hippocrates, Galen, Ibn Sīnā, John of Gaddesden, and Gilbertus Anglicus.[8] Such a citation indicates the reputation of Bernard's work, only recently being reconsidered in greater detail by scholars such as Luke Demaitre and Linda E. Voigts.[9] The *Lilium* is an extensive treatise on disease aetiology, diagnostics, personal case studies, and treatment recipes. The text was widely disseminated during the medieval period; the Latin text of the *Lilium* is extant in over 50 manuscripts and several printed editions.[10] Furthermore, it was translated into a range of vernaculars, including Hebrew, French, Spanish, and Irish. As Chaucer's statement indicates, the *Lilium* is connected with a wider tradition of medical writings during the medieval period. For instance, Bernard of Gordon is referenced three times in the surgeon John Arderne's treatise *Fistula in ano* for his anatomical description of urethral fistula, his method of diagnosing haemorrhoids, and his recipe for treating tenesmus.[11] The *Lilium medicinae* was

---

[6] Harrison *et al.* (2015); Bald's eyesalve is contained in *Bald's Leechbook*, British Library Royal MS. 12 D XVII.
[7] Harrison *et al.* (2016).
[8] Benson (1980: 30).
[9] Demaitre (1980, 2013); Voigts (2003: 233–252; 2004: 149–160).
[10] Demaitre (1980: 51).
[11] Power (1910/1968: 14, 55, 73).

cited in John of Gaddesden's *Rosa medicinae*, which has been described by Tony Hunt as being 'heavily indebted' to the *Lilium* and 'an inferior imitation of the *Lilium*' by Paul Diepgen.[12]

The *Lilium* was part of the curriculum at the University of Montpellier in the 14th century. It was required reading at the University of Vienna in 1520, and the last known printing occurred as late as 1697 in a Spanish translation.[13] A page of a 1542 (Paris) printed edition presented by Luke Demaitre in his study of medieval medicine is covered with extensive notes by a late 16th-century reader.[14] The multiple manuscript copies, several languages, and many printed versions (all occurring over a 400-year span of time), as well as the active engagement with the material demonstrated in some editions, are all evidence of the text's long-standing and widespread interest even into the early modern period. Although there are multiple witnesses in Latin, there is only one extant translation in English, the *Lylye of Medicynes*, which survives in a 15th-century manuscript, Oxford Bodleian Library MS Ashmole 1505.

The presentation of the recipes in the *Lylye* follows a standard format. Each recipe begins with an indication of what type of remedy it is, such as syrup, drink, or plaster, and usually when it should be used (at the beginning, middle, or end of an illness). A list of diverse ingredients with specific quantities is then given. The ingredient list is followed by instructions for preparation of the medicine, such as boil, dry, powder, infuse, and how long it will take to prepare the medicine. Some medications, such as *pelotys* (pills), could be made in advance, dried in 'shadowe' (cool, dry conditions) and then prepared with milk or wine when they were ready to be used. Other, more complicated medicines, such as *triacle*, required dozens of different ingredients and a preparation time of many weeks. The final step in such recipes is administration of the treatment to the patient. Treatments, like medicinal preparations, also vary in the length of time. A simple fever, such as *effimera*, was expected to be of such short duration that it was cured in a single day, whereas a patient with a broken leg could expect to be confined to bed for at least 40 days with continual monitoring and intervention by the doctor. Some ointments and plasters were changed multiple times during the day and night, and depending on the severity of the illness, some recipes admonish the physician to *wakeþ* (be vigilant).

There are 360 recipes in the text prefaced with *Rx*, but every chapter gives lengthy lists of additional materials and ingredient combinations which are to be used at the reader's discretion according to what is available or the patient's

---

[12] Hunt (1990: 26); Diepgen is quoted in Demaitre (1980: 59).
[13] Demaitre (2013: 30).
[14] Demaitre (2013: xi).

particular symptoms. Purgative medicines are the most used remedy in the text. Of the nearly 6000 ingredients referenced in the *Lylye*, about 85 percent are individual ingredient names, such as borage, vinegar, and wine, while 9 percent are compound medicines, like *triacle*, and 6 percent are products of alchemical processes, such as mercury and white lead. One examination of the *Corpus Hippocraticum* found that of the 3000 references to medicinal products, the most frequently occurring are wine, honey, and vinegar.[15] A similar distribution is noted in the *Lylye*, which is not surprising considering the value of such elements as the basic vehicles (or solvents) for nearly every medical preparation, as well as their antiseptic properties. In the *Lylye*, various species of *Plantago* are administered for a number of conditions, including wounds, skin infections, general oral diseases, abscesses in the gums, burns (by water or fire), nail infections, nosebleed, digestive complaints, diarrhoea, liver problems, ruptured cornea, respiratory conditions (cough, throat infections), vomiting blood, kidney stones, and blood in the urine. The following will present four recipes from the Middle English *Lylye*[16] used to treat cutaneous wounds (and one additional recipe for a mouthwash). Ingredients from the genus *Plantago* are highlighted in bold along with the preparation method (maceration) and combination with wine or vinegar, which will be discussed later.

The first recipe is from Book 1, *De vulneribus*, which deals with all manner of wounds, including cuts from swords and other cutaneous wounds, bruises, open head wounds, broken bones, and wounds in nerves, muscles, vasculature, and organs. The following recipe is for a cutaneous wound that has turned into an ulcer, which the text defines as red, purulent, and foul (fol. 38r).

> And ȝif it be vlcus wiþ hete oþer by enchesoun of hete or by enchesoun of brennynge of fuyre oþer of hoote watere oþer of þe sunne, þan enonyte þe place wiþ popileon and wex and vnguentum citrinum. Oþer make an oynement of þese þyngis: **muscilago psillij**, camphore, and sandali, and rosis, and **succo** portulace, **plantago**, papaueris, and coriandri. (fol. 40r)

The next three recipes come from a chapter (Book 1, *De apostematibus calidis generatis per viam adustionis*) that deals with skin swellings/abscesses, lesions, infected wounds, carbuncles, and erysipelas. Symptoms listed in the text include broken skin, purulence, itching, foul smell, great heat and/or inflammation, aching, pricking and burning sensations, redness, yellowness, ulceration, and black crusts, which are all evidence of infection. The first recipe appears under the

---

[15] Hunt (1990: 2).
[16] Currently I am preparing an edition of the *Lylye of Medicynes*. The edited excerpts from the *Lylye* presented here are my own.

subhead *De formica miliari*, which is described as pustules with heat that move from place to place on the skin and sometimes produce ulcers (fol. 27v). Note that forms of *Plantago* are used in all stages of the treatment.

> In þe first bygynnynge, ley vppon þe place lactuca **ygrounden** and portulaca, **muscilaginis psillij**. And in þe myddel, ordeum and brede þat is branny and **plantayne** and ryndis of maligranati. And towarde þe ende, sal and nitrum and ruwe and cucumer asinini, and medle hem wiþ childis pisse and **iuse of planteyne**. For in al þese þynges þe mater is venymous. Grete studye and grete cautele þou most do þerto, as it were in igne persico. (fol. 27v)

The following two recipes are from the subsection titled *De herisipula, antrace, carbunculo, et sacri ignis*. The first recipe is to be prepared at the beginning of the condition.

> In þe first bygynnynge or þe skyn be to broke, þan in þe place is grete heete and akynge and prickynge and redenesse and ӡelownesse, þan make colde þe place wiþ a sponge wette in colde water oþer wiþ lactuca and portulaca and nenifar and leuys of a whyte vyne and **planteyn** and barlich. **Grynde** oon of alle þese oþer alle and ley þeron. (fols. 25v–26r)

The second recipe concerns ulcerated wounds or a severe skin infection that is not responding to the first treatment.

> Kytte a pome garnet in þe myddel and **boyle** in **vynegre** and þan **grinde** hyt and lay hyt þeron and about ley bole and **vynegre** and after þat ne lay þou þerto no moyste þynge. For woundes ne mow noӡt be cured but hy be first made drye. Þerfore, lay þerto colde þynges and stiptica wiþ resolutyues and openynge.
>
> Þynges þat falliþ herfore beþ þese: **plantago**, virga pastoris, portulaca, coriandrum, cerusa, plumbum vstum, bolus, acacia, opium, nitrum, sal, sulphure, nux antiqua vnctuosa, oleum rosarum, cucumeri asinini, fel hircinum, piper, panis cum multo furfure, ciclamen, galle, lentes, alumen, granata acetosa, vua passa, fficus, camphore, cera alba, **vinum ponticum**. Þe leche schal be diligent and alle þese þynges or some and **seþe hem in vynegre and grynde hem and ley þeron** and remeue þe plastre 3 tymes a day and nyӡte. (fol. 26r)

Finally, as an aside due to its connection with the above two recipes from *De herisipula, antrace, carbunculo, et sacri ignis*, a recipe found in Book 3, *De pascionibus oris,* is to be used for oral complaints related to carbuncles or 'wild fire' (possibly erysipelas):

> ȝiff it be carbunculus oþer wilde fuyre, make hym a gargarisme wiþ þe **iuse of plantayn**, coriandre, morelle in **wyn of maligranata** flach. (fol. 125v)

In another treatment given in the *Lylye* for pustules and festers, a lengthy list of ingredients is given with the statement 'ȝif þou ne knowyst noȝt what þou schalt do, vse þis oynement', which suggests that when all else fails, use as many ingredients as possible (fol. 38r). The second recipe from *De herisipula, antrace, carbunculo, et sacri ignis* given here, with its lengthy and varied ingredient list, does seem to indicate this idea of multiplying ingredients when desperate for a cure. However, using the scientific literature around *Plantago* and its healing properties, it may be possible to show that more methodology is contained in these prescriptions than first appears. Although the theoretical model of medieval medicine (humoral theory) has long been proved incorrect, the medicines and herbs used to treat illness certainly have quantifiable effects or, as suggested in the *Lylye*, the medicines 'sleiþ and curiþ' (fol. 26v).

There are about 240 species of *Plantago*.[17] The genus has a long history in herbal medicine from ancient times to the present day. Dioscorides and others used it as a cure-all.[18] The 'Nine Herbs Charm' in the *Lacnunga* describes *Plantago* as the *wyrta modor* ('mother of herbs').[19] Hildegard of Bingen's *Physica* states to mix it with wine or honey as a treatment for gout. It is also cited as a useful application for insect stings and as an antidote to love spells.[20] It was favoured by John Arderne as a surgical salve and remedy against inflammation in his treatise, *Fistula in ano*.[21] The 16th-century master of the London Company of Barber-Surgeons, Thomas Gale, noted the anti-inflammatory properties of 'plantaginis' and used it in a 'speciall plaster for all kyndes of vlcerations, as well of the legges'; the recipe occurs in a section that references treatments for the leg ulcers of Henry VIII.[22] A 2006 survey of ethnoveterinary medicine in British Columbia identified the

---

[17] Kuiper and Bos (1992: 4). Some sources say up to 260 species (such as Efrayim and Zohar 2008: 242).
[18] Efrayim and Zohar (2008: 242).
[19] Cameron (2006: 144, 192); the *Lacnunga* is contained in British Library MS Harley 585.
[20] Throop (1998: 53).
[21] Power (1910/1968: 117).
[22] Gale (1563: fols. 54, 66, second book of the *Antidotarie*).

practice of applying the leaves of *Plantago major* L. to abscesses, wounds, and skin rashes of horses.[23] Furthermore, the Norwegian and Swedish term for *Plantago major* is *groblad,* meaning 'healing leaves'.[24] Similarly, a 2014 study into the efficacy of *Plantago major* to combat skin pathogens called it 'Nature's Band-aid' for its effectiveness as a remedy for cuts, burns, and insect stings.[25] The herb has been in continual usage from ancient times. There are nearly 40 references to it in the *Lylye,* often in association with wound care or infectious conditions. Anecdotal evidence in folkloric medicine has existed for centuries, but several scientific studies have provided more substantial evidence of its healing properties.

Plantago has been associated with many beneficial properties, including antibiotic, antiviral, antioxidant, anti-inflammatory, anticancer, wound healing, and immuno-enhancing effects. A search of the PubMed database was performed for the years 2000 to 2015. The search was restricted to studies testing the antimicrobial, wound healing, or immune effects of *Plantago major* or *Plantago lanceolata* L., as these two species are particularly associated with these activities in the literature. Although *psillij* is in the genus *Plantago*, and is present in some of the medieval recipes given previously as examples, it was not examined in this instance. The search was also restricted to studies published in the English language. Review articles were excluded from the search. Eleven studies were selected for further enquiry based on their relevance to the search criteria.[26] Kováč *et al.* (2014) tested *P. lanceolata*; Nostro *et al.* (2000) tested *P. lanceolata* and other herbal remedies; Chiang *et al.* (2003), Thomé *et al.* (2012), and Nilson *et al.* (2014) tested *P. major* and other herbal remedies, while the rest of the studies tested only *P. major*. These studies cover a range of topics and results, but, in summary, there is evidence that extracts from *P. major* and *P. lanceolata* demonstrate wound healing properties and antimicrobial activity with potential significance for future research. Figure 1 shows a summary of the distribution of the surveyed studies in four general categories.

To return to the previous medieval recipes from the *Lylye*, which mentioned a variety of symptoms including open skin wounds, broken skin, symptoms of infection, and ulcerated tissue, the following will specifically consider two studies that evaluated the efficacy of *P. major* and *P. lanceolata* for wound healing (without infecting the wounds) and then will briefly consider investigations into the

---

[23] Lans *et al.* (2006).
[24] Samuelsen (2000: 2).
[25] Nilson *et al.* (2014).
[26] Chiang *et al.* (2002); Chiang *et al.* (2003); Gomez-Flores *et al.* (2000); Hetland *et al.* (2000); Karima *et al.* (2015); Kováč *et al.* (2014); Metiner *et al.* (2012); Nilson *et al.* (2014); Nostro *et al.* (2000); Thomé *et al.* (2012); Türel *et al.* (2009).

Author	Remedy tested	Year	Method	Anti-microbial	Wound healing	Anti-inflammatory	Immuno-enhancing
Karima et al.	P. major	2015	in vitro	X			
Kováč et al.	P. lanceolata	2014	in vivo		X		
Nilson et al.	P. major and other herbal remedies	2014	in vitro	X			
Metiner et al.	P. major	2012	in vitro	X			
Thomé et al.	P. major and other herbal remedies	2012	in vivo		X		
Türel et al.	P. major	2009	in vivo			X	
Chiang et al.	P. major and other herbal remedies	2003	in vitro	X (antiviral)		X	X
Chiang et al.	P. major	2002	in vitro	X (antiviral)			
Gomez-Flores et al.	P. major	2000	in vitro				X
Hetland et al.	P. major	2000	in vivo	X			X
Nostro et al.	P. lanceolata and other herbal remedies	2000	in vitro	X			

Figure 1. Summary of the distribution of selected studies

antibacterial activities of the two species, as efficient wound healing and infection prevention are two parts of one whole in the recovery process.

Thomé et al. (2012) performed an *in vivo* mouse (Swiss line) study using *P. major* compared with a water-treated control group, another herbal remedy (*Siparuna guianensis* Aubl.), and a commercially available ointment used in Brazil. *P. major* leaves (100 g) were collected in Minas Gerais State (Brazil), washed with clean control at room temperature, dried, ground to a fine powder and added to a hydro-alcoholic solution (70 percent). After maceration (48 hours), the extract was filtered, freeze-dried (lyophilized), and incorporated into a lanolin and paraffin ointment base at a 10 percent (w/w) concentration.[27] Mutagenicity tests showed that *P. major* was not mutagenic. An incision wound was made in the cervical dorsal area of the mice. They observed that 'reduction of the wound area occurred earlier' in the *P. major* cohort and that '*P. major* extract effectively stimulated wound-healing processes'.[28] There was also more efficient formation of neoepithelium in the *P. major* cohort (and the other herbal extract, *S. guianensis*) compared with the commercially available ointment. The authors state that *P. major* is a 'promising candidate for the treatment of wounds'.[29]

Kováč et al. (2014) performed an *in vivo* rat (Sprague-Dawley) study using a water extract of *P. lanceolata*, which was prepared by adding 10 g of dried *P. lanceolata* leaves to 100 ml of boiling distilled water and allowing it to infuse for 10 minutes at room temperature. Two concentrations were tested—the original concentration obtained by extraction (10 percent) and a 10-times-diluted concentration (1 percent). Two excisional wounds and one incisional wound were made on the back of the rats. In the control group, nothing was applied (untreated wounds), and in the negative control group, the wounds were treated with sterile water. In the two experimental groups, either the high (10 percent) or low concentration (1 percent) solutions were applied. Compared with the untreated control group and water-treated group, wounds treated with both the high and low concentrations of *P. lanceolata* showed significantly improved wound closure and significantly increased tensile strength due to an increase in extracellular matrix proteins. Notably, healing rates of both wound types were significantly increased after treatment with the high concentration of *P. lanceolata*.[30]

The studies above investigated the effect of certain *Plantago* species on wound healing without infection. The following will consider evidence for antimicrobial activity. Some early *in vitro* studies from the 1960s to the late 1980s

---

[27] Thomé *et al.* (2012: 1380).
[28] Thomé *et al.* (2012: 1382, 1385).
[29] Thomé *et al.* (2012: 1379).
[30] Kováč *et al.* (2014: 122).

cited by the European Medicines Agency (2011) indicate that pressed juice and aqueous extracts of *P. lanceolata* showed antibacterial effects against *S. aureus, Streptococcus β-hemolyticus, Proteus vulgaris, Salmonella, Shigella, Pseudomonas aeruginosa, Klebsiella pneumoniae, Bacillus subtilis,* and *Micrococcus flavus.*[31] These microbes are responsible for conditions such as cutaneous infections, hospital infections (MRSA, surgical wound infections), respiratory infections, Strep throat, urinary tract infections, vomiting and diarrhoea, burn infections, pneumonias, and other opportunistic infections. Nostro *et al.* (2000) performed a comparative study of six medicinal plants and found that while *P. lanceolata* showed inhibitory activity, it was not as pronounced as other plants in the study (namely, *Helichrysum italicum* [Roth] G.Don and *Nepeta cataria* L. [Labiatae]).[32] In contrast, Orhan *et al.* (2002) did not observe antibacterial or antifungal effects when ethanolic extracts of *P. lanceolata* were tested against *Escherichia coli, Proteus mirabilis, Enterococcus faecalis, Acinetobacter baumannii, P. aeruginosa, S. aureus, Streptococcus pneumoniae, Candida albicans, Candida kruzei,* and *Candida parapsilosis.*[33]

Metiner *et al.* (2012) tested acetone and ethyl alcohol extracts of *P. major* leaves against *Bacillus cereus, B. subtilis, S. aureus, Staphylococcus epidermidis, E. coli, K. pneumoniae, P. aeruginosa, P. mirabilis,* and *Salmonella enteritidis.* They found that the ethyl alcohol extract exhibited antibacterial activity against *E. coli* and *B. cereus,* while the acetone extract was effective on all the species in the different experimental concentrations. While the authors do not recommend *P. major* as an antibiotic on its own, they conclude that 'it contributes to prevent the formation of infection in wounds with its remarkable antibacterial effectiveness'.[34] Along those lines, Hetland *et al.* (2000) isolated a pectin polysaccharide from the leaves of *P. major* and found that it had a protective effect against systemic *S. pneumoniae* in mice due to stimulation of the innate immune system.[35] Nilson *et al.* (2014) found that *P. major* extracts showed efficacy against *S. aureus,* but not *P. aeruginosa.* They suggest that the antimicrobial compounds in medicinal plants may be more effective against gram-positive bacteria.[36] Finally, in testing the efficacy of extracts from *P. major* leaves in combination with the antibiotic gentamicin, Karima *et al.* (2015) found 'a significant synergistic effect' against *P. aeruginosa, S. aureus, B. cereus, P. mirabilis,* and *Salmonella typhimurium.*[37] The selection of studies briefly

---

[31] European Medicines Agency (2011: 16).
[32] Nostro *et al.* (2000: 383–384).
[33] European Medicines Agency (2011: 16).
[34] Metiner *et al.* (2012: 505).
[35] Hetland *et al.* (2000: 348).
[36] Nilson *et al.* (2014).
[37] Karima *et al.* (2015: 63).

surveyed here shows a variable range of results in regard to antimicrobial activity and presents an intriguing suggestion that *Plantago* spp. may function best as a partner with antibiotics or with other medicinal plants. This concept of ingredient synergy also correlates with Harrison *et al.*'s study of Bald's eyesalve, which was most effective in the combination of ingredients rather than as isolated individual agents. The co-occurrence of the genus *Plantago* with other medicinal plants, such as pomegranate (which occurs in three of the five medieval recipes given here as examples), may be worth exploring in greater detail.

Finally, aucubin is one of the biologically active compounds of *Plantago*, and some studies have reported 'antibiotic activity' for aucubin isolates.[38] Notably, it is stored in the leaves as an inactive precursor and is enzymatically activated when the leaves are ground up or crushed. The selected studies, including the two wound healing studies previously described, prepared extracts from the plant material using alcohol, water, and maceration techniques, concurring with the medieval method of preparation. In the *Lylye*, *Plantago* is often soaked, boiled and ground up with vinegar, water, or wine (as in the recipes given as examples). The best method of extracting aucubin from the leaves is a consideration for future research. The European Medicines Agency suggests that the method of drying (and the temperature change) may impact extraction, as opposed to working with fresh leaves. Also, in the medieval and modern examples presented here, the leaves are often boiled, whereas, for example, Youyou Tu found that the active ingredient for her antimalarial treatment was extracted after soaking the leaves in cold water as opposed to boiling.[39]

This discussion has been a brief enquiry into the potential efficacy of a few recipes contained in a specific medieval medical text to treat infected wounds in light of selected scientific investigations. Underlying this enquiry is the idea that remedies in the 'old books' of medical history may be used as inspiration for novel pathways in present-day research against infectious conditions. Channelling historical medical texts into new drug discovery is only possible through interdisciplinary collaboration. It requires close working relationships, shared convictions, openness to challenges, and knowledge exchange between experts in medieval medicine, manuscript studies, microbiology, chemistry, pharmacology, and data science. More interdisciplinary research, utilising knowledge from both the arts and sciences, is necessary to gain a fuller understanding of the antimicrobial and healing powers of these ingredients. This research will provide insights into whether these medieval remedies were simply placebos, or actual

---

[38] European Medicines Agency (2011: 16).
[39] Thank you to Freya Harrison for suggesting the importance of aucubin (personal communication).

antibiotics being used long before the advent of the modern science of wound care and infection control.

Acknowledgements

This paper was written for the 2014 conference when I was in the second year of my PhD programme. It was revised in 2015 and again in 2017. Thank you to Christina Lee, Nicola Royan, Freya Harrison, and Steve Diggle for commenting on early drafts.

Bibliography

Manuscripts
London British Library MS Harley 3698
London British Library MS Sloane 334
London British Library MS Sloane 512
London British Library MS Sloane 3096
Oxford Bodleian Library MS Ashmole 1505

Other Sources
Benson, L. (ed.) 1987. *The Riverside Chaucer*, 3rd ed. Oxford: Oxford University Press.
Cameron, M. 2006. *Anglo-Saxon Medicine*. Cambridge: Cambridge University Press.
Chen, L., Todd, R., Kiehlbauch, J., Walters, M., Kallen, A. 2017. Notes from the field: Pan-resistant New Delhi metallo-beta-lactamase-producing *Klebsiella pneumoniae*—Washoe County, Nevada, 2016. *Morbidity and Mortality Weekly Report* 66: 33.
Chiang, L. C., Chiang, W., Chang, M. Y., Ng, L. T., Lin, C. C. 2002. Antiviral activity of *Plantago major* extracts and related compounds *in vitro*. *Antiviral Research* 55: 53–62.
Chiang, L. C., Chiang, W., Chang, M.Y., Lin, C. C. 2003. *In vitro* cytotoxic, antiviral, and immunomodulatory effects of *Plantago major* and *Plantago asiatica*. *American Journal of Chinese Medicine* 31(2): 225–234.
Cockayne, O. 1864–1866. *Leechdoms, wortcunning and starcraft: being a collection of documents, for the most part never before printed, illustrating the history of science before the Norman conquest* (Rolls series 35th, 3 vols). London: Longman, Green, Longman, Roberts, and Green.
Connelly, E. 2017. My written books of surgery in the Englishe Tonge: The Barber-Surgeons Guild of London and the *Lylye of Medicynes*. *Manuscript Studies: A Journal of the Schoenberg Institute for Manuscript Studies* 2.2.

Costeo, G. and Mongio, G. P. (eds) 1595. *Avicennae Canon Medicinae*. Venice: Apud Juntas. Available at Google eBooks, <http://books.google.co.uk>.

Demaitre, L. 1980. *Doctor Bernard of Gordon*. Toronto: Pontifical Institute of Mediaeval Studies.

Demaitre, L. 2013. *Medieval Medicine: The Art of Healing from Head to Toe*. Santa Barbara (CA): Praeger.

Efrayim, L. and Zohar, A. 2008. *Practical Materia Medica of the Medieval Eastern Mediterranean According to the Cairo Genizah*. Leiden: Brill.

European Medicines Agency, Committee on Herbal Medicinal Products 2011. Assessment report on *Plantago lanceolata* L., folium, EMA/HMPC/437859/2010, viewed 27 August 2017 at <http://www.ema.europa.eu/docs/en_GB/document_library/Herbal_-_HMPC_assessment_report/2012/02/WC500123351.pdf>.

Gale, T. 1563. *Certaine Workes of Chirurgerie*. London: Rouland Hall, Boston Medical Library Collection, viewed 27 August 2017, <www.archive.org>.

Getz, F. 1991. *Healing and Society in Medieval England: A Middle English Translation of the Pharmaceutical Writings of Gilbertus Anglicus*. Madison: University of Wisconsin Press.

Gomez-Flores, R., Calderon, C. L., Scheibel, L. W., Tamez-Guerra, P., Rodriguez-Padilla, C., Tamez-Guerra, R., Weber, R. J. 2000. Immunoenhancing properties of *Plantago major* leaf extract. *Phytotherapy Research* 14(8): 617–622.

Harrison, F., Roberts, A. E. L., Gabrilska, R., Rumbaugh, K. P., Lee, C., and Diggle, S. P. 2015. A 1,000-year-old antimicrobial remedy with antistaphylococcal activity. *mBio* 6(4), viewed August 2017, <http://mbio.asm.org/content/6/4/e01129-15>.

Harrison, F., Gabrilska, R., Azimi, S., Rumbaugh, K. P., Lee, C., and Diggle, S. P. 2016. The potential of medieval 'ancientbiotics' in the treatment of chronic biofilm infection. Presentation to the 2016 Annual Conference of the Microbiology Society, Liverpool (UK).

Hetland, G., Samuelsen, A. B., Løvik, M., Paulsen, B. S., Aaberge, I. S., Groeng, E. -C., Michaelsen, T. E. 2000. Protective effect of *Plantago major* L. Pectin polysaccharide against systemic *Streptococcus pneumoniae* infection in mice. *Scandinavian Journal of Immunology* 52(4): 348–355.

Hunt, T. 1990. *Popular Medicine in Thirteenth-Century England*. Cambridge: D. S. Brewer.

Karima, S., Farida, S., Mihoub, Z. M. 2015. Antioxidant and antimicrobial activities of *Plantago major*. *International Journal of Pharmacy and Pharmaceutical Sciences* 7(5): 58–64.

Kew Medicinal Plant Names Services, viewed 27 August 2017, <http://mpns.kew.org>.

Kováč, I., Ďurkáč, J., Hollý, M., Jakubčová, K., Perželová, V., Mučaji, P., Švajdlenka, E., Sabol, F., Legáth, J., Belák, J., Smetana, K. Jr, Gál, P. 2014. *Plantago lanceolata* L. water extract induces transition of fibroblasts into myofibroblasts and increases tensile strength of healing skin wounds. *Journal of Pharmacy and Pharmacology* 67: 117–125.

Kuiper, P. J. C. and Bos, M. (eds) 1992. *Plantago: A Multidisciplinary Study* (Ecological Studies 89). Berlin: Springer-Verlag.

Lans, C., Turner, N., Brauer, G., Lourenco, G., Georges, K. 2006. Ethnoveterinary medicines used for horses in Trinidad and in British Columbia, Canada. *Journal of Ethnobiology and Ethnomedicine* 2(31).

Metiner, K., Ozkan, O., Ak, S. 2012. Antibacterial effects of ethanol and acetone extract of *Plantago major* L. on gram positive and gram negative bacteria. *Kafkas Üniversitesi Veteriner Fakültesi Dergisi* 18(3): 503–505.

Nilson, S., Gendron, F., Bellegarde, J., McKenna, B., Louie, D., Manson, G., Alphonse, H. 2014. Preliminary scientific investigation of the effectiveness of the medicinal plants *Plantago major* and *Achillea millefolium* against the bacteria *Pseudomonas aeruginosa* and *Staphylococcus aureus* in partnership with indigenous elders. *Global Journal of Research on Medicinal Plants and Indigenous Medicine* 3(11): 402–415.

Nobelprize.org. 2015. Press Release 2015-10-05: Nobel Prize in Physiology or Medicine <https://www.nobelprize.org/nobel_prizes/medicine/laureates/2015/press.html>.

Opus lilium medicinae 1559. Lyon: Apud Gulielmum Rouillium. Available at Google eBooks, <http://books.google.co.uk>.

Nostro, A., Germanò, M. P., D'angelo, V., Marino, A., Cannatelli, M. A. 2000. Extraction methods and bioautography for evaluation of medicinal plant antimicrobial activity. *Letters in Applied Microbiology* 30: 379–384.

Power, D. (ed.) 1910/1968. *Treatises of Fistula in Ano, Haemorrhoids, and Clysters by John Arderne from an Early Fifteenth-Century Manuscript Translation* (EETS Original Series 139). Oxford: EETS.

Practica seu Lilium Medicinae 1497. Venice: Johannes and Gregorius de Gregoriis for Benedictus Fontana. Available at Bayerische StaatsBibliothek, <http://www.bsb-muenchen.de/index.php>.

Review on Antimicrobial Resistance. 2014, December 11. Antimicrobial resistance: Tackling a crisis for the future health and wealth of nations, viewed 25 August 2017, <https://amr-review.org/Publications.html>.

Review on Antimicrobial Resistance. 2016, May 19. Tackling drug-resistant infections globally: Final report and recommendations, viewed August 2017, <https://amr-review.org/Publications.html>.

Robbins, R. H. 1970. Medical manuscripts in Middle English. *Speculum* 45(3): 393–415.

Samuelsen, A. B. 2000. The traditional uses, chemical constituents and biological activities of *Plantago major* L.: A review. *Journal of Ethnopharmacology* 71(1–2): 1–21.

Thomé, R. G., dos Santos, H. B., dos Santos, F. V., da Silva Oliveira, R. J., de Camargos, L. F., Pereira, M. N., Longatti, T. R., Souto, C. M., Franco, C. S., de Oliveira Aquino Schüffner, R., Ribeiro, R. I. 2012. Evaluation of healing wound and genotoxicity potentials from extracts hydroalcoholic of *Plantago major* and *Siparuna guianensis*. *Experimental Biology and Medicine* 237(12): 1379–1386.

Throop, P. (trans., ed.) 1998. *Hildegard Von Bingen's Physica: The Complete English Translation of Her Classic Work on Health and Healing*. Rochester (VT): Healing Arts Press.

Tu, Y. 2011. The discovery of artemisinin (qinghaosu) and gifts from Chinese medicine. *Nature Medicine* 17: 1217-1220, doi:10.1038/nm.2471.

Türel, I., Özbek, H., Erten, R., Öner, A. C., Cengiz, N., Yilmaz, O. 2009. Hepatoprotective and anti-inflammatory activities of *Plantago major* L. *Indian Journal of Pharmacology* 41(3): 120–124.

Voigts, L. E. 2003. The master of the king's stillatories, in J. Stratford (ed.), *The Lancastrian Court: Proceedings of the 2001 Harlaxton Symposium*: 233–252. Donington: Shaun Tyas.

Voigts, L. E. 2004. Takamiya MS 60 and the Middle English text of Bernard of Gordon's *De Pronosticis*, in T. Matsuda, R.A. Linenthal, and J. Scahill (eds), *The Medieval Book and a Modern Collector*: 149–160. Cambridge: D. S. Brewer.

World Health Organization. 2017, September 20. The world is running out of antibiotics, viewed September 2017 <http://www.who.int/mediacentre/news/releases/2017/running-out-antibiotics/en/>.

World Health Organization. 2016, September. Antimicrobial resistance fact sheet, viewed August 2017, <http://www.who.int/mediacentre/factsheets/fs194/en/>.

Miserum spectaculum, horrendus fetor, aspectus horrendus: 'Syphilis' in Strasbourg at the Turn of the 16th Century

Christoph Wieselhuber

In 1495, in the aftermath of the battle of Fornovo in Italy (5 July), soldiers of the French king, Charles VIII, began to complain about swellings on their skin and later about pain with increasing intensity. One of the first physicians on site was Alessandro Benedetti from Venice, who described the symptoms of the ailment as follows: 'The entire body is so repulsive to look at and the suffering is so great, especially at night, that this sickness is even more horrifying than incurable leprosy or elephantiasis, and it can be fatal.'[1] Benedetti called the ailment the 'French Sickness'. His colleague Girolamo Fracastoro introduced the term 'syphilis' in his work 'Hieronymi Fracastorii Syphilidis, sive Morbi Gallici, Libri tres, ad Petrum Bembum' (first half of the 16th century).[2] In 1496, Strasbourg (estimated inhabitants: over 20,000)[3] was one of the first imperial cities where a disease with the same symptoms was reported. The preacher of the Strasbourg Cathedral, Johannes Geiler von Kaysersberg (1445–1510), called it 'blattern' (pox), presumably because of the tumorous lesions that came with it. From a medical point of view, to construct a connection of both outbreaks is problematic at best and is a matter of continuous debate in the scientific community. The question of whether terms from the Early Modern Period, such as *blattern*, *pocken* and *syphilis*, merely have similar symptoms and a similar etiopathology or if they all are associated with the same disease may never be answered.[4] However, in our context it is not of great importance, as social responses to all of these sexually transmitted illnesses are comparable. The limited medical knowledge of the time prohibited any further differentiation of the subject. Our interest here is not the ailments themselves, but the social standing of those afflicted by them, whatever those ailments may be, as perceived and evaluated by Johannes Geiler, who was 'the prince of the pulpit in

---

*The citation in the title by: Geiler (1518b: fol. 35v).
[1] Quétel (1992: 10).
[2] Eatough (1984).
[3] Voltmer (2008: 196).
[4] Jütte (2005: 141); Keil (1999: 380); Walter (2003: 172).

the late 15th and early 16th centuries' and one of the most influential citizens of Strasbourg outside of the city council.[5]

Geiler first addressed the city council about the problem of the people infected with this new disease in the winter of 1496. In a letter, Geiler suggested removing infected people from outside the city from the hospital to a private house.[6] The text suggests that a citizen called Wilhelm Böcklin would be willing to provide such an accommodation. This measure was necessary in the preacher's view in order to alleviate some of the pressure upon the hospital and to open it up again for those entitled to its services: the inhabitants of Strasbourg.[7] Furthermore, Geiler recommended that a carer should be appointed to tend to all those 'ellenden mönschen' (miserable people) suffering from the disease.[8] Despite appearances, the theologian's motivations were not unworldly. He realised the practical problems and economic strain that his suggestions to the council would create: the carer would have to be paid from the city treasury, and at least food and clothing would have to be provided for the carer. Therefore, he proposed to expel the strangers from the city in case of food shortage or—in the best case—when the weather improved.[9] This remark remains a little bit of a mystery since it could be interpreted in a sarcastic sense, as a criticism of the council's social politics, which was a recurring theme in Geiler's sermons.

As Rita Voltmer pointed out, there was no intention to provide any medical treatment for those infected, citizens or otherwise.[10] The authorities and medical practitioners were at a loss as to how to address this crisis. It appears that the city council even tried to close the city gates to people who came to Strasbourg seeking help. Geiler's letter evidently spurred the authorities to action, and the proposed 'Blatternhaus' became a reality (1502/03).[11] Some time later the preacher made the new situation public by speaking about it from the cathedral pulpit.[12] His description gives us a glimpse into the conditions in the *Blatternhaus*: sick people were wasting away under terrible circumstances; they were fed by the hospital,

---

[5] Steinmetz (2001: 9); for further reading about Geiler, I recommend Voltmer (2005).
[6] The fact that the illness was not named specifically in the letter is explained by Rita Voltmer. All parties involved knew about the outbreak. It was, therefore, not necessary to refer to it separately (Voltmer 1996: 425).
[7] Dacheux (1882: 109–10).
[8] Dacheux (1882: 109).
[9] Dacheux (1882: 110).
[10] Voltmer (1996: 425).
[11] Pfleger (1918: 162).
[12] Voltmer dates this sermon to 1 January 1497 (Voltmer 1996: 426); Pfleger, on the other hand, presumes that Geiler spoke about the Blatternhaus in 1503 (Pfleger 1918: 166).

but not cared for in a medical sense.[13] Even citizens from the city were moved from the hospital to the *Blatternhaus* when they showed the symptoms. Almost half of the patients in the *Blatternhaus* were not from Strasbourg, which means that the sickness had spread to even the more sparsely populated regions around the city.

Furthermore, over 90 percent of city dwellers in the late medieval period resided in small towns.[14] Therefore, it is reasonable to assume that not only people from rural areas sought help in Strasbourg. Most of the infected inhabitants of Strasbourg were servants.[15] However, this is by no means an indication of a correlation between social status and probability of infection. It is more than likely that those who could be treated in the seclusion of their homes gladly took this opportunity. Geiler mentioned this point almost casually and did not try to estimate the number of unreported cases.[16]

Despite the fact that Geiler regarded the outbreak of *blattern* in Strasbourg as divine punishment, he consulted with physicians to obtain a better understanding of the sickness.[17] All of his efforts in dealing with this crisis were aimed at helping the afflicted and not condemning and isolating them.[18] It is not clear whether the sexual transmission of the pathogen was known to Geiler, but it is likely that he was aware of it because most texts about the disease at the turn of the 16th century

---

[13] Geiler (1518b: fol. 35ᵛ).
[14] Engel and Jacob (2006: 8).
[15] Geiler (1518b: fol. 35ᵛ).
[16] Geiler (1521b: fol. 35ᵛ); Voltmer (1996: 426).
[17] Geiler (1515: fol. CXLIXʳ [numbered as CLIXʳ]); Voltmer (1996: 427–428).
[18] Bauer (1989: 182–183): ‚[. . .] Darumb sollen die blotterechten nit ußgeschlossen werden und also verlassen das sie nachts uff den gassen zu todt mochten erfrieren / deshalb das sie nackend hungerig und dar zu todtsiech sind [. . .] / Darumb so ist es ein grosse hertikeit die weder vor got noch der werlt verantwurdet mag werden ich hore das es in anderen stetten nit geschehe [. . .]'. Geiler (1518b: fol. XXXVᵛ): Vestrum ergo erit fratres charissimi / manus extendere / et liberaliter eis elemosynam impe[n]dere / non parce. Qui enim parce seminat / parce et meret. Quilibet iuxta suam facultatem / omnes tamen aliquid / et nemo nihil prestet. [. . .] Qui multum habet multum prestet. Nobilis nobiliter / et liberaliter. Qui miles est / aut doctor quibus aurum licet deferre / non argentum offerant sed aurum / non plapbardos / sed florenos: similiter et exorum uxores. Et hi qui libenter essent milites / aut femine quae vellent habere milites in maritos, omnes aurum offerant. Sed et hi qui divites sunt / similiter multa dent. Certi estis de fidelitate administratorum / egoipse oculum adhibeo, ut in usus illorum exulum dstribuatur elemosyna per vos prestanda / precipue autem sacerdotes et perlati ecclesiarum et monasteriorum sint liberalissimi.' Geiler (1518b: fol. XXXVIʳ): 'Omnes aliquid offera[n]t puero Jesu p[ro]pter nos hodie circu[m]ciso. Circumcidamus [et] superflua in pecuniis propter eum qui propter nos circumcisus est in prepuciis.'

suggest some connection to the sexual act.¹⁹ This does not mean, however, that there was a heuristic approach to the epidemic. Syphilis, as an abstract plague, was perceived as divine punishment for 'houbetsünden' (like murder, unchastity, paederasty), and a cure was only possible by redemption.²⁰ Geiler's explanation for the disease was a theological one, so the best prevention of infection was an unassailable lifestyle. Humans became infected not *through* sexual activity, but *because of* sexual activity engaged in against the moral standards of the Christian community.²¹ A compilation of Geiler's 1504 sermons on sexual activity was published in 1517:

> Jetzund so hab ich für mich genummen / die blattern die da seind am heimlichen ort / an der scham wann die selben blattern die seind sorglich wann man zeugt sie gar vngern vnd man schampt sich ir gar übel / also seind die blattern / das ist die sünd die an dem heimlichen ort verbracht werden / das seind die sünd vnküscheit / die seind sorglich / wan man sie selten recht zögt vnd clarlich daruon beichtet / vnnd es seind diese hienach Bubenketzer Kuketzer Frauwenketzer Fründschender Junckfrauwenschender Raub Eebruch [. . .] Einfaltigklich unküscheit.²²

> (Now I will talk about the *blattern* in a secret place: the pubic areas. You admit to them unwillingly and you are ashamed because of them. The *blattern* are a sign of the sins of a secret place, sins like unchastity, which you seldom admit to have committed. Unchastity includes the sins of *Bubenketzer* [paederasts, homosexuals], *Kuketzer* [those who commit bestiality], *Frauwenketzer* [rapists], *Fründschender* [those committing sexual violence against a friend], *Junkfrauwenschender* [men who violate a woman or girl and refuse to marry her], . . . robbery, adultery).

The disease Geiler described was—from his point of view—a direct response to capital sins. In 1505, Geiler compared the *blattern* in Strasbourg with the leprosy in Egypt described in the Old Testament in his sermons about 'blattern at the mouth'.²³ He argues that when the lesions of the illness appear next to the mouth, they mark the physical spot of the victim's transgressions, and indicate sins

---

[19] Quétel (1992: 22).
[20] Thoma (2009: 140).
[21] Voltmer (1996: 440–441).
[22] Geiler (1517: fols. VII^r–VIII^r).
[23] Exodus 9:8–10.

committed by the mouth: lying, gossiping and so on.[24] He declares that sexual sins are to be atoned for likewise. Herein, he follows the tradition of church doctrine in the later Middle Ages by interpreting catastrophes from an eschatological point of view as punishment for violating the Ten Commandments. He commented, in agreement with Benedetti, that *blattern*/syphilis—despite its curability—is worse than leprosy.[25] However, as Lev Mordechai Thoma observed, Geiler's suggestion of a connection between the Egyptian plague of leprosy with the sin of unchastity seems to have been his original idea.[26] The preacher interpreted the symptoms of *blattern*/syphilis developing at the genitals as stigmata marking people who committed capital sins like rape, robbery, adultery or homosexuality. The physical disfigurement is accompanied by an equally disgusting image of the person's character traits which Geiler created in his sermons. But this image of the punished sinner remains a stereotype in Geiler's sermons and is never transferred to real people infected with the disease. This strategy is compelling, since Geiler always aimed to return the sinner to the flock. An exception is the mention of two sodomites in a sermon who were burned in Strasbourg in 1506. He even identified them by name and profession: Hieronymus and a bottle maker whose name is not given.[27] This break with anonymity is at first glance puzzling. However, since the burning of these two men accused of sodomy was a public event, it would have made no sense to shroud their identity. Instead, he used this example as a starting point for the subject, a point with which all of Strasbourg was most likely familiar. Thoma suggests that this particular sermon, edited by Johannes Pauli in 1517, seven years after Geiler's death, is a compilation of three different sermon texts.[28] As the case may be, the sermon compilation 'summarises Geiler's thoughts' overall about sodomy.[29] In his foreword, Pauli states that the preacher of the Cathedral of Strasbourg spoke about 'blattern in a secret place' in the year 1506. The editor pictured himself as someone picking up the breadcrumbs of the actual preaching of the subject.[30] The image of breadcrumbs can be interpreted in two ways: either

---

[24] Geiler (1518a: fol. II^v): 'Da verhengt gott zehe[n] blage[n] und straffe uber das Egipten landt / als in dem anderen buch Moisi Exodi an dem .ix. eigentlich geschribe[n] stot / und under andere[n] blagen / mit denen der her den kunig un[d] die Egipter strafft / das ware[n] t blatere[n].'

[25] Geiler (1518b: fol. 35^v): 'presertim in pudensis cosque urit, ut longe minus turpe sit et tolerabilius esse leprosum quam tali scabie infectum, solo hoc dempto, quod hec curabilis, lepra autem non.'

[26] Thoma (2009: 141).

[27] Geiler (1517: fol. VII^r).

[28] Thoma (2009: 138).

[29] Thoma (2009: 140) (my translation).

[30] Geiler (1517: fol. VII^r).

it is an understatement to show the editor's unworthiness to write down Geiler's words—a conventional topos in literature at the time—or Pauli used this picture to demonstrate that Geiler's sermons (or parts of them) on the subject had been collected like breadcrumbs. Despite the fact that none of the edited sermons may represent Geiler's direct words (which is almost always a problem when working with medieval sermons), Johannes Pauli's trustworthiness in conveying Geiler's ideas and perspectives has been reestablished in the scientific community after Peter Wickgram's devastating judgment was dominant for the better part of a century.[31] However, the question remains if the focus on *blattern* at the genitals as a result of sodomy was Geiler's sincere belief or a construction suggested by the character compilation made by Pauli. After all, unchastity can have many faces, as Geiler himself pointed out, and so can the reason for divine punishment.[32]

Despite his conviction that repentance must come before the body can be healed by a doctor's hand, the preacher was faced with the harsh reality of the disease.[33] In his 21 articles to the city council in 1500, Geiler again lamented the predicament of those infected with the condition and complained about their lying on the streets, where they were certain to freeze to death.[34] However, living with the disease inside the city walls produced another social reaction in the course of time: halfheartedness. After the first wave of terror ebbed away, the disfigured victims of the disease were almost taken for granted.[35] To counteract this public lethargy, Geiler used emblematic techniques in the form of biblical references to illustrate misbehaviour on society's part, a common and effective tool in many sermon texts.[36] The sick beggar Lazarus became a symbol of the individual suffering from *blattern*, lying in front of the rich man's house, shoved into the background of the public mind by society's ability to adapt their conscience in the course of time.[37] Geiler perceived the sick individual primarily as a victim, in contrast to his theoretical elaborations. Although the punishment manifests itself in the infected person, it is Christian society and humankind as a whole who are being

---

[31] Bauer (1994: 571–573).

[32] Geiler (1517: fol. VIIr–VIIIr).

[33] Bauer (1989: 13): 'Sitt einmol das gar dick lipliche kranckheit uß dem gebresten der sele einen ursprunck hat. so hatt der babst durch ein offen ußgetruckt gebot eym ieglichen lib artzet geboten das er keinem siechen lipliche arzenye gebe ee das er in verman zesuchen den geistlichen artzt. das ist der bichter. Darumb sint wie es nutz wer das in allen spitalen. oder gotzhusern ein gesatz gemacht wurd das kein krancker do uff genommen wurd der nit bereitet wer zebichten.'

[34] Bauer (1989: 182).

[35] Voltmer (1996: 431).

[36] Ramatschi (1934: 177).

[37] Geiler (1522: Part 3, fol. XXXX^v); Luke 16:19–31.

judged by the Almighty. Geiler's two-sided strategy in dealing with the medical crisis demanded, on one hand, repentance on a cultural level, while protecting the individual in the generalised mass, and, on the other hand, the acknowledgement of social responsibility by the society. In Geiler's point of view, it was his task as self-appointed 'Wächter auf dem Turm' (guardian on the tower) to lead the people of Strasbourg through this moral crisis:

> Etliche sind die ougen [/] die selben synd die / die da me weißheit und clarer verstentnuß haben denn andere menschen / für die sye sollend sehen / wie der wechter uff dem turn / der für alle die / die in der stat sind [/] sicht.[38]

> (There are many people who are the eyes because they possess more wisdom and a mind more clear than other people. They should watch out like the guardian on the tower who stands watch for all people in the city.)

More precisely, he puts it in his sermon text 'Arbore Humana' (preached in 1495 or 1497):

> Der wechter uff dem thurn die weil es brint un[d] knaßlet / so hört er nit uff zu schreien und sturme[n] / zu dem minsten das das feuer nit weiter umb sich eß.[39]

> (When there is fire in the city, the guardian on the tower keeps shouting and calling to prevent the fire from spreading even further.)

Geiler regarded the outbreak of *blattern* as punishment on a societal scale, because the whole society was involved in living with and combating the disease. Even the uninfected had to repent by helping those who contracted the illness, either on a personal level or in an economic sense. To avoid any stigmatisation of the victims of *blattern* and society's tendency to encapsulate itself from those infected on a physical and moral level, Geiler preached against the illness by creating the image of a faceless sinner, an unassailable bogeyman, whenever possible. The fact that the preacher's intent was never to cast those infected out of society becomes clear when Geiler was dealing with the victims on a personal level in his sermons. In this context, helping is always paramount in Geiler's texts; even people from outside the city of Strasbourg are considered for help, at least shortly after the outbreak.

---

[38] Bauer (1995: 724).
[39] Geiler (1521a: fol. CIII^v); Voltmer (2005: 31).

Geiler's motif for this twin-track strategy seems clear. Indifference towards those who need help is against the God-given order of society. Every man has a specific place in the divine order on earth:

> Das geistlicher frid ist [. . .]. Ein Stille / ein heitere der ordenung / da alle ding in dir rüwig unnd stil seind. [. . .] Als da ist / wann der Ammeister sitzet / da er sitzen sol / deß gleichen der Stettmeister / und also ein yeglicher an seiner stat. Item da man laßt in friden die handtwerckßlüt / den Schuhmacher / de[n] Schneide[r] / de[n] Brotbecker in seiner ruh und stille. Wa her kummen krieg / dann das einer den anderen von seiner stat stosset / und einer den andern bei dem har danne zücht / und einer hat das der ander haben solt / da ist nit gottes frid / wiewol ordenung da ist / so ist doch kein stille da.[40]

> (Spiritual peace is a tranquility in which all things are repentant and still. This means that the Ammeister [title of the mayor of Strasbourg] is in his place as is the Stettmeister [a three-month rotating office similar to the mayor in Strasbourg] and are all the others. Leave the craftsmen, the shoe maker, the tailor, the baker in peace to be penitent and still. In wartime one is expelling the other from his post, one is pulling the hair of the other, one has in his possession something that belongs to the other. That is not God's peace. There may be order, but there is no tranquillity.)

Geiler is referring to the 'corpus mysticum', the principle of the order of Christian society. It is on the one hand a rigid construct where social change is hard or even impossible; on the other hand, it is also a guarantor for most people to be included in this 'corpus'. The citizen's right to exist as part of this system is independent from factors like legal status or sex.[41] The inequality of individuals is in fact one of the arguments to legitimate their existence, for, as Geiler notes, a body in which all organs have the same function cannot survive. The image of the 'community body' demonstrates Geiler's view of society: if one or more organs is sick, it is the body as a whole that has sinned and must repent.

Geiler believed that particularly in a crisis situation, like a threatening ailment, this societal system is in danger of becoming eroded. In this case, however, the social aspects of the differentiation are limited to the nursing capacities and the medical possibilities of the social environment the patient is bound by. But public perception is, naturally, focused on those sick individuals who define the

---

[40] Geiler (1515: fol. CXIII^r); Voltmer (2008: 203–204).
[41] Voltmer (2006: 93).

townscape and who are reliant on the city's willingness to help: mostly aliens and the lower classes. As Geiler pointed out, people who could afford to be cared for in their homes would not seek the help of the *Blatternhaus*, but neither would they be eligible for it.

Yet a purely social imbalance is not the catalyst of the disturbance of the natural order that Geiler is worried about. It is rather the sheer scale of this human catastrophe and the fear of further spreading of the disease. In 1500, Strasbourg closed its doors to aliens who were suspected of begging. Two years later, inhabitants of the city diagnosed with *blattern* were no longer allowed in public gatherings and taverns.[42] However, they were allowed to beg inside the city walls, which reinforced the public image of the disease.[43] Geiler endeavoured to contain the outbreak, based on his theological understanding of the disease, by urging the community of the city to lead a morally impeccable life. But, in doing so, he risked a stigmatisation of those infected. Therefore, Geiler tried to keep the threat abstract by never attaching the aspect of sin to the *Blatternhaus* or its inhabitants. Geiler walked a tightrope to accomplish these conflicting goals: saving society, while protecting the individual. The seeming inconsistency associated with this strategy reflects our own confusion when dealing with one of the questions most often left unanswered in medieval studies: is there a mandatory connection between illness and sin?[44] Perhaps we should rephrase the question: *What* is the connection between illness and sin?

Bibliography

Bauer, G. (ed.) 1989. *Johannes Geiler von Kaysersberg. Sämtliche Werke, Erster Teil: Die deutschen Schriften, Erste Abteilung: Die zu Geilers Lebzeiten erschienenen Schriften, Band 1* (Ausgaben deutscher Literatur des XV. bis XVIII. Jahrhunderts). Berlin: Walter de Gruyter.

Bauer, G. 1994. Johannes Geiler von Kaysersberg: Ein Problemfall für Drucker, Herausgeber, Verleger, Wissenschaft und Wissenschaftsförderung. *Daphnis* 23: 559–589.

Bauer, G. (ed.) 1995. *Johannes Geiler von Kaysersberg. Sämtliche Werke, Erster Teil: Die deutschen Schriften, Erste Abteilung: Die zu Geilers Lebzeiten erschienenen Schriften, Band 3.* (Ausgaben deutscher Literatur des XV. bis XVIII. Jahrhunderts). Berlin: Walter de Gruyter.

---

[42] Voltmer (1996: 433).
[43] Voltmer (1996: 436).
[44] Vollmer (2011: 263).

Dacheux, L. (ed.) 1882/1965. *Die ältesten Schriften Geilers von Kaysersberg. XXI Artikel—Briefe—Todtenbüchlein—Beichtspiegel—Seelenheil—Sendtbrieff—Bilger.* Amsterdam: Editions Rodopi.

Eatough, G. (ed.) 1984. *Fracastoro's Syphilis. Introduction, Text, Translation and Notes with a computer-generated word index* (ARCA Classical and Medieval Texts, Papers and Monographs 12). Liverpool: Francis Cairns.

Engel, E. and Jacob, F. -D. 2006. *Städtisches Leben im Mittelalter. Schriftquellen und Bildzeugnisse.* Cologne: Böhlau.

Geiler, J.; J. Pauli (ed.) 1515. *Das Euangelibuch Das buoch der Ewangelien durch das gantz iar, Mitt Predig vnd vßlegunge[n] durch . . . Doctor Johannes geiler vo[n] Keisersperg . . . vß seinnem mund vo[n] wort zu wort geschribe[n] . . . .* Strasbourg: Johannes Grüninger.

Geiler, J.; J. Pauli (ed.) 1517. *Die brösamlin doct. Keiserspergs vffgelesen vo[n] Frater Johan[n] Paulin barfuser orde[n]s. Vnd sagt vo[n] de[n] funfftzehen Hymelschen staffelen die Maria vff gestigen ist. vn[d] ga[n]tz von de[n] vier Leuwengeschrei. Auch von dem Wa[n]nenkromer der Kauflüt sunderlich hüpsche matery bei. xii predige[n].* Strasbourg: Johannes Grüninger.

Geiler, J.; J. Pauli (ed.) 1518a. *Das buch der sünden des munds. Von dem hochgelerten Doctor Keysersperg / die er nent die blatren am mund davon er xxix predigen und leeren gethon hat.* Strasbourg: Johannes Grüninger.

Geiler, J.; P. Wickgram (ed.) 1518b. *Sermones et varii tractatus Keiserspergii iam recens excuse.* Strasbourg: Johannes Grüninger.

Geiler, J. 1521a. *Das buoch Arbore humana. Von dem menschlichen baum / Geprediget von dem hochgelerten Doctor Johannes Keysersperg / darin geschicklich und in gottes lob zuo lernen ist / des holtzmeyers des dotz / frölich zu warten / Einem yeden menschen nütz und guot.* Strasbourg: Johannes Grüninger.

Geiler, J.; P. Wickgram (ed.) 1521b. *Sermones et varij Tractatus Kaiserspergii iam recens excusi. quorum Indicem versa pallega videbis. Endecasyllabum Otthomari Luscini. . . . In laudem operum doctissimi Keiserspergij.* [Argentina]: Johannes Grüninger.

Geiler, J.; H. Wessmer (ed.) 1522. *Doctor keiserszbergs Postill. Vber die fyer Euangelia durchs jor / samt dem Quadragesimal / vnd von ettlichen Heyligen / newlich vßgangen* (4 parts). Strasbourg: Johann Schott.

Jütte, R. 2005. Die 'Syphilis' im frühneuzeitlichen Köln, in T. Deres (ed.) *Krank—gesund. 2000 Jahre Krankheit und Gesundheit in Köln*: 140–153. Cologne: Kölnisches Stadtmuseum.

Keil, G. 1999. 'Syphilis'. *Lexikon des Mittelalters* 8: 380–381.

Pfleger, L. 1918. Das Auftreten der Syphilis in Straßburg, Geiler von Kaysersberg und der Kult des hl. Fiakrius. *Zeitschrift für die Geschichte des Oberrheins* 72: 153–173.

Quétel, C., Braddock, J., and Pike, B. (trans.) 1992. *History of Syphilis.* Baltimore: Johns Hopkins University Press.

Ramatschi, P. 1934. Geiler von Kaysersberg 'Der Has im Pfeffer': Ein Beispiel emblematischer Predigtweise. *Theologie und Glaube* 26: 176–191.

Steinmetz, D.C. 2001. Johannes Geiler von Kaysersberg (1445–1510). Pastoral care and human responsibility, in D.C. Steinmetz, *Reformers in the Wings: From Geiler von Kaysersberg to Theodore Beza*: 9–14. Oxford: Oxford University Press.

Thoma, L. M. 2009. 'Das seind die sünd der vnküscheit'. Eine Fallstudie zum Umgang mit der Sodomie in der Predigt des ausgehenden Mittelalters. Die 'Brösamlin' Johannes Geilers von Kaysersberg, in L. M. Thoma and S. Limbeck (eds), *'Die Sünde, der sich der tiuvel schamet in der helle'. Homosexualität in der Kultur des Mittelalters und der frühen Neuzeit*: 137–153. Ostfildern: Thorbecke.

Vollmer, M. 2011. Sünde—Krankheit—'väterliche Züchtigung': Sünden als Ursache von Krankheiten vom Mittelalter bis in die Frühe Neuzeit, in A. Classen (ed.), *Religion und Gesundheit. Der heilkundliche Diskurs im 16. Jahrhundert* (Theophrastus Paracelsus Studien): 261–286. Berlin: Walter de Gruyter.

Voltmer, R. 1996. Praesidium et pater pauperum, pustulatorum praecipua salus. Johannes Geiler von Kaysersberg und die Syphilis in Straßburg (1496–1509), in F. Burgard, C. Cluse, and A. Haverkampf (eds), *Liber Amicorum necnon et Amicarum für Alfred Heit. Beiträge zur mittelalterlichen Geschichte und geschichtlichen Landeskunde* (Trierer Historische Forschungen 28): 413–444. Trier: Trierer Historische Forschungen.

Voltmer, R. 2005. *Wie der Wächter auf dem Turm. Ein Prediger und seine Stadt. Johannes Geiler von Kaysersberg (1445-1510) und Straßburg* (Beiträge zur Landes- und Kulturgeschichte 4). Trier: Porta Alba.

Voltmer, R. 2006. Zwischen polit-theologischen Konzepten, obrigkeitlichen Normsetzungen und städtischem Alltag: Die Vorschläge des Straßburger Münsterpredigers Johannes Geiler von Kaysersberg zur Reform des städtischen Armenwesens, in S. Schmidt und J. Aspelmeier (eds), *Norm und Praxis der Armenfürsorge in Spätmittelalter und früher Neuzeit* (Vierteljahresschrift für Sozial- und Wirtschaftsgeschichte. Beihefte): 189. Stuttgart: Steiner.

Voltmer, R. 2008. 'Die fueß an dem leichnam der christenhait / seind die hantwercks leüt. arbaiter / baŭleüt / und das gemayn volck. . .'. Die Straßburger Unterschichten im polit-theologischen System des Johannes Geiler von Kaysersberg, in S. Schmitt and S. Klapp (eds), *Städtische Gesellschaft und Kirche im Spätmittelalter* (Kolloquium Dhaun 2004, Geschichtliche Landeskunde): 62. Stuttgart: Steiner.

Walter, T. 2003. Die Syphilis als astrologische Katastrophe: Frühe medizinische Fachtexte zur 'Franzosenkrankheit', in D. Groh, M. Kempe, and F. Mauelshagen (eds), *Naturkatastrophen. Beiträge zu ihrer Deutung, Wahrnehmung und Darstellung in Text und Bild von der Antike bis ins 20. Jahrhundert* (Literatur und Anthropologie 13): 165–186. Tübingen: Narr.